Medically Fragile Training Manual

Geri Hernandez

Medically Fragile Training Manual

Tate Publishing & *Enterprises*

Published by Tate Publishing & Enterprises, LLC
127 E. Trade Center Terrace | Mustang, Oklahoma 73064 USA
1.888.361.9473 | www.tatepublishing.com

Tate Publishing is committed to excellence in the publishing industry. The company reflects the philosophy established by the founders, based on Psalm 68:11,
"The Lord gave the word and great was the company of those who published it."

Cover design by Blake Brasor
Interior design by Nathan Harmony

Published in the United States of America

ISBN: 978-1-61566-258-6
1. Medical: Caregiver
2. Medical Education & Training
09.11.09

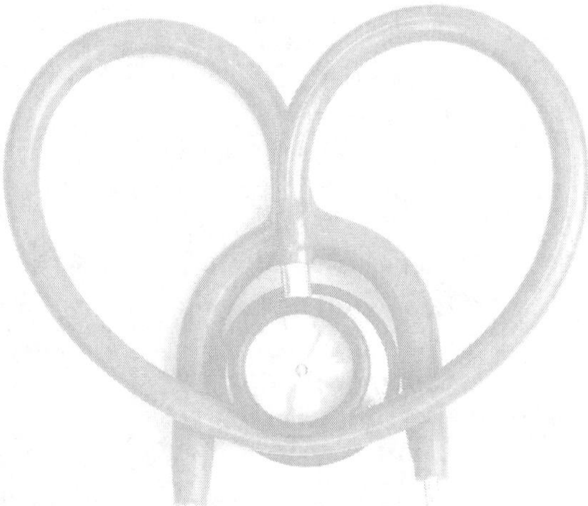

Table of Contents

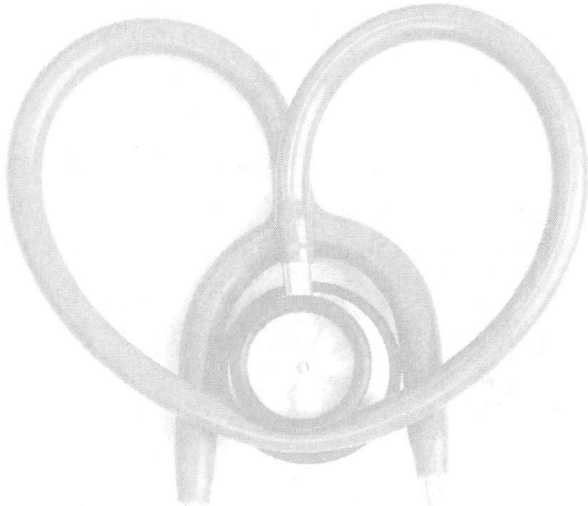

Disclaimer

The clinical treatments described and recommended in this training manual are based on research and consultation with nursing, medical, and legal authorities. To the best of the author's knowledge, these procedures reflect currently accepted practice. Nevertheless, they can't be considered absolute and universal recommendations. For individual applications, all recommendations must be considered in light of the patient's clinical condition. The author disclaims any responsibility for any adverse effects resulting from the suggested procedures, from any undetected errors, or from the reader's misunderstanding of the text.

The use of the manual is not intended to replace the advice of a doctor. The manual is intended to help people make better health care decisions and take a greater responsibility for their own health. You expressly acknowledge and agree that the authors, suppliers, licensees, and publisher are not responsible for the results of your decisions resulting from the use of the manual, including, but not limited to, your choosing to seek or not to seek professional medical care or your choosing or not choosing specific treatment based on the manual.

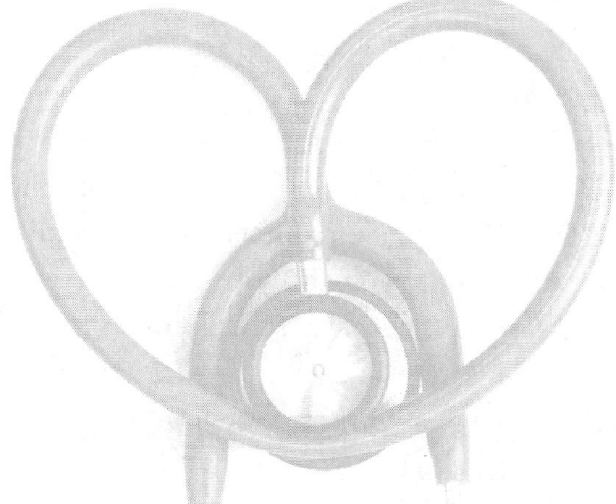

What is Medically Fragile?

In 1989, the passage of Assembly Bill (AB) 2268 (Bates) allowed foster family homes to provide services to technology-dependent children in a home environment. Prior law had prohibited residential facilities licensed by Department of Social Services, Community Care Licensing Division (CCLD), from providing more than incidental medical care to children. However, advances in medical science were saving the lives of children who would not have survived a decade earlier left them dependent on medical technology. Many of these children became long-term "boarders" in a hospital or other health care institutions because there was no place for them to live after their medical conditions stabilized.

The new law permitted children who are court dependent and had special health care needs to be placed in licensed foster family homes under specific conditions. It also mandated an individualized health care plan outlining a child's medical needs and the licensee's responsibilities. The health care plan team must also appoint a health care professional to monitor the medical services provided to the child by trained foster parents for whom the nursing scope of practice laws are waived.

Two more recent pieces of legislation build on AB 2268. As of January 1, 1992, AB 760 (Bates) permitted children with special health care needs to reside in licensed, small-family homes. This law defined the term "specialized foster care homes" to include small-family homes as well as licensed foster family homes. The law also expanded the definition of children to be served to include children with developmental disabilities who are receiving services and case management from a regional center.

AB 636 (Bates), effective October 1, 1993, expanded the definition of "specialized foster care home" to include family homes certified by a foster family agency. Further, AB 636 changed the definition of "children with special health care needs" to include medically fragile children.

Who Are the Children with Special Health Care Needs?

To be defined as having "special health care needs," a child must have a need for specialized in-home health care based upon one or both of the following:

Medical conditions that require dependency upon one or more of the following:

- Enteral feeding tube
- Total parenteral feeding
- Cardiorespiratory monitoring
- Intravenous therapy
- Ventilator
- Oxygen support
- Urinary catheterization
- Renal Dialysis
- Ministrations imposed by tracheotomy, colostomy, ileostomy, or other medical or surgical procedures.
- Special medication regimens, including injection, and intravenous medication.

Also, any condition that can rapidly deteriorate resulting in permanent injury or death. These children are referred to as "medically fragile."

Typically, medically fragile children are infants or young children (under two and a half years of age) who are prone to rehospitalization. The foster parent must be trained to recognize the onset of deterioration should it persist, even if all medical procedures and ministrations are correctly performed. The following are a few examples of conditions that often, but certainly not always, qualify a child as medically fragile.

- Prenatal exposure to drugs and/or alcohol
- Congenital or hereditary defects such as spina bifida, sickle cell anemia, cystic fibrosis, heart defects.
- Burns
- Epilepsy
- Bronchopulmonary dysplasia
- Failure to thrive
- HIV positive and symptomatic
- Prematurity

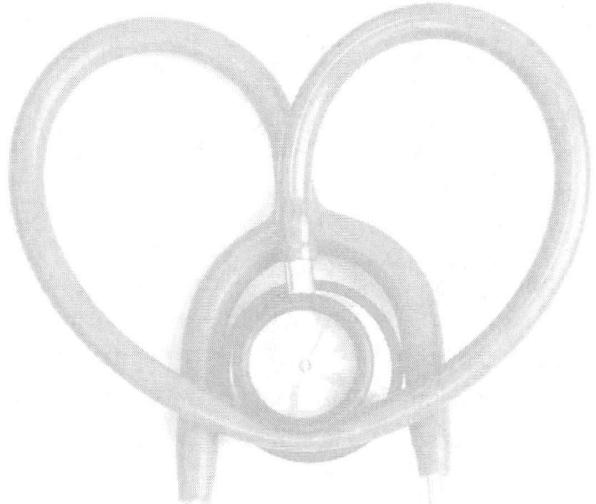

Individualized Health Care Plans

A team of people create an individualized health care plan. The child's primary care physician or designee, county social worker or regional center caseworker, and the in-home monitor of the child's individualized health care plan must be on the team. The individualized health care plan team may include: a public health nurse; representatives from the disability prevention program; parents, if reunification is a goal; and the prospective specialized licensee.

The licensee may not accept a child with special health care needs unless the licensee has obtained an individualized health care plan.

Individualized health care plan: The plan may be a hospital discharge plan but shall include the following information:

- The name, address, and phone number of the physician or other health care professional responsible for monitoring the consumer's ongoing health care.
- Written verification by the consumer's individualized health care plan team, identifying the specialized in-home health care appropriately administered by a responsible adult trained by a health care professional.
- Arrangements for in-home health support services if required.
- Identification of any available and funded medical services that are to be provided to the consumer in the home, which may include assistance from registered nurses, licensed vocational nurses, public health nurses, physical therapists, and respite care workers.
- The individualized health care plan can be combined with the consumer's needs and service plan (IFSP) as long as all information required by both plans is included. The individualized health care plan must contain clearly stated instructions regarding what the foster parent is required to do.
- The consumer must have current Individual Planning Program (IPP) within thirty days of placement.
- Description of consumer's service needs, ambulatory status, medical needs, and special dietary requirements.

- Information regarding individual abilities and preferences (likes and dislikes).
- Current and historical data regarding aggressive and/or dangerous behavior toward self or others.
- Identified needs for training and treatment.

The individualized health care plan is a critical document, as the required information is the primary means for licensing to monitor the health and safety of children with special health care needs in licensed facilities. The plan must contain clearly stated instructions regarding what the foster parent is supposed to do. This information may be located in other records such as the child's IPP (for regional center clients) or a hospital discharge plan.

The appropriate number of hours of on-site supervision and monitoring and the appropriate number of hours of off-site supervision and monitoring needed to be provided by the nurse specified in Section 88069.1(a)(1), AB 2268.

The individualized health care plan for each child with special health care needs shall be updated at least every six months or sooner if the needs of the child change.

Individualized Health Care Plan (Sample)

Name: Child's Name Updated: Needs to be updated every six months or as necessary

Problem #1 Alteration in feeding mode and behaviors R/T G-tube placement

Secondary to failure to thrive and severe prematurity

Goal/objective:

1. Maintain tube placement
2. Maintain calorie intake via G-tube/NGT to support nutrition
3. Increase feedings to a degree that will support total nutritional needs for optimum growth and development

Interventions:

1. Caregivers will follow orders prescribed by MD for feeding program
2. Document results of feedings to assess need to change or readiness to learn new skills
3. Follow outlined program consistently to promote maximum effectiveness and to see need for any alterations in program plan
4. Evaluation: It is best to do an evaluation when you get the baby for placement and then update the evaluation within six months or sooner as needed. This is a good way to keep track of progress and is a helpful tool. The nurse assigned to your home will help you with the problems, goals, and interventions. Each child should have at least three problems that you are working on, and more, if needed. For more examples, see sample forms and checklist.

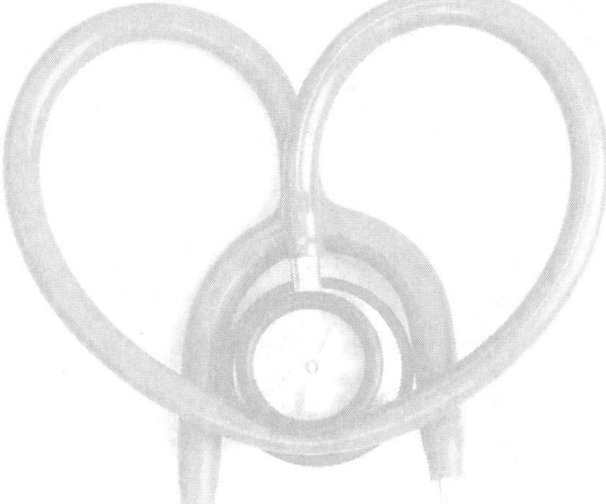

Common Medical Diagnoses for the Medically Fragile Infant

Birth Defects

Cleft Palate

The word cleft means a gap or split between two things. A cleft lip is a split in the upper lip. This can happen on one or two sides of the lip, creating a wider opening into the nose. A cleft palate is a split in the roof of the mouth. This leaves a hole between the nose and the mouth. Sometimes a cleft lip and cleft palate occur together in the same child.

Cleft lip and cleft palate are birth defects, which mean they happen while a baby is developing inside his or her mother. Normally, the mouth and nose of a baby develop between the first six and twelve weeks of growth. In some babies, parts of the lips and roof of the mouth don't grow together. Because the lips and the palate develop separately, it's possible to have cleft lip, cleft palate, or both.

We don't always know why a particular baby has cleft lip or cleft palate. Sometimes the condition runs in families. Other times, cleft palate is part of a syndrome, meaning there are birth defects in other body parts too. Most of the time, however, the cause of the cleft is unknown and cannot be prevented.

A baby with cleft lip or cleft palate may have problems eating. This can be a big problem, especially for a newborn baby. Fortunately, there are feeding specialists and special baby bottles that can help.

Children with cleft palates can have hearing loss, dental problems, and speech problems. Therefore, children with cleft palates should have their ears and hearing checked once or twice a year, see an orthodontist, and work with speech therapists to counteract these problems.

Treating cleft lip or cleft palate takes a team of different types of specialists. This team includes a plastic surgeon, a speech language pathologist, an orthodontist, an otolaryngologist (a doctor trained in ear, nose, and throat problems), an oral surgeon, a dentist, a geneticist, a social worker, a psychologist, an audiologist, and other health care specialists. Because there are so many different people for a child to see, the team has a coordinator who works with the parents and foster parents to help organize everything.

Cleft lip is usually repaired by the time a baby is three to six months old. During surgery on the cleft lip, the doctor closes the gap in the lip and corrects the nostril. A person who has a cleft lip repaired as an infant will have a scar on the lip under the nose.

Cleft palate is usually repaired at age nine to twelve months. During surgery on cleft palate, doctors close the hole between the roof of the mouth and the nose and reconnect the muscles in the soft palate.

Spina Bifida

Myelomeningocele, the most common form of spina bifida, is characterized by incomplete formation of the spinal column in which a thin sac protrudes on the back and contains a portion of the spinal cord, meninges, and spinal fluid. Alpha-fetoprotein levels in amniotic fluid can detect the defect, which occurs in about one in one thousand live births. The location of the defect determines the severity of the symptoms.

Potential complications include paralysis, joint deformities, meningitis, and lack of bladder or bowel control. Treatment involves surgery, antibiotic administration, physical therapy, and bladder and bowel retraining. Many children are able to walk with the use of crutches or braces.

Arnold-Chiari syndrome: Arnold-Chiari syndrome, an elongation or tongue-like downward projection of the cerebellum and medulla through the foramen magnum into the spinal canal, occurs in all infants with the myelomeningocele form of spina bifida. Hydrocephalus often accompanies the defect, resulting from impaired drainage of cerebrospinal fluid. Besides the signs and symptoms of hydrocephalus, other indications of Arnold-Chiari syndrome include neck rigidity, noisy respirations, irritability, vomiting, a weak sucking reflex, and hyperextension of the neck.

Treatment requires surgical placement of a shunt like that used in hydrocephalus. Surgical decompression of the cerebellar tonsils at the foramen magnum sometimes is indicated.

All infants with myelomeningocele have Arnold-Chiari syndrome; however, only about 10 percent of these infants become symptomatic. Hydrocephalus aggravates this problem.

Spina bifida is a birth defect that involves the incomplete development of the spinal cord or its coverings. The term spina bifida comes from Latin and literally means split or open spine. Spina bifida occurs at the end of the first month of pregnancy when the two sides of the embryo's spine fail to join together, leaving an open area. In some cases, the spinal cord or other membranes may push through this opening in the embryo's back. The condition can typically be detected before a baby is born and treated right away. The causes of spina bifida are largely unknown. Some evidence suggests that genes may be involved, but in most cases, there is no familial connection.

There are two forms of spina bifida: spina bifida occulta and spina bifida manifesta.

- Spina bifida occulta is the mildest form of spina bifida (occulta means hidden). Most children with this type of defect never have any health problems. The spinal cord is often unaffected.
- Spina bifida manifesta includes two types of spina bifida: meningocele and myelomeningocele.

Meningocele involves the meninges, the membranes responsible for covering and protecting the brain and spinal cord. If the meninges push through the hole in the vertebrae (the small, ringlike bones that make up the spinal column), the sac is called a meningocele.

Myelomeningocele is the most severe form of spina bifida. It occurs when the meninges push through the hole in the back and the spinal cord also pushes though. Most babies who are born with this type of spina bifida also have hydrocephalus, an accumulation of fluid in and around the brain. Because of the abnormal development of and damage to the spinal cord, a child with the myelomeningocele form of spina bifida typically has some paralysis. The degree of paralysis largely depends on where the opening occurs in the spine. The higher the opening is on the back, the more severe the paralysis tends to be.

Children with spina bifida often have problems with bowel and bladder control, and some may have attention deficit hyperactivity disorder (ADHD) or other learning difficulties such as hand-eye coordination problems.

Babies who are born with spina bifida occulta often have no outward signs or symptoms. The spinal cord does not protrude through the skin, although a patch of hair, a birthmark, or a dimple may be present on the skin over the lower spine. But in other forms of the disease, there are obvious signs. Babies who are born with the meningocele form of the disease have a sac filled with fluid that is visible on the back. The sac is often covered by a thin layer of skin and can range in size from the dimensions of a grape to those of a grapefruit.

Babies who are born with myelomeningocele also have a saclike mass that bulges from the back, but a layer of skin may not always cover it. In some cases, the nerves of the spinal cord may be exposed. A baby who also has hydrocephalus will have an enlarged head, the result of excess fluid and pressure inside the skull.

Children with spina bifida occulta usually need no treatment. In cases of spina bifida manifesta, the treatment largely depends on the type of spina bifida a child has and how severe it is. A child with the meningocele form of the disease usually has an operation during infancy in which doctors push the meninges back and close the hole in the vertebrae. Many children with this type of spina bifida have no other health problems down the road, unless there is nerve tissue involved with the sac.

Babies born with the myelomeningocele form of the condition need more immediate attention and typically have surgery within the first one to two days of their lives. During this first surgery, doctors typically push the spine back into the vertebrae and close the hole to prevent infection and protect the spine. A baby who also has hydrocephalus will need an operation to place a shunt in the brain. The shunt is a thin tube that helps to relieve pressure on the brain by draining and diverting extra fluid. In addition, some children need subsequent surgeries to manage problems with the feet, hips, or spine.

The location of the gap in the back often dictates what kind of adaptive aids or equipment that a child with myelomeningocele will need down the line. Children with a gap high on the spinal column and more extensive paralysis will often need to use a wheelchair to move around, whereas those with a gap lower on the back may be able to use crutches, leg braces, or walkers.

Foster parents of children with spina bifida will receive support from a medical team that may include several doctors (such as neurosurgeons, urologists, orthopedic surgeons, rehabilitation specialists, and general pediatricians), a nurse practitioner, physical and occupational therapists, and a social worker. The goal is to create a lifestyle for the child and family in which the disability interferes as little as possible with normal, everyday activities.

Circulatory

Common Heart Defects

Common types of congenital heart defects, which can affect any part of the heart or its surrounding structures, include:

- Aortic Stenosis: In aortic stenosis, the aortic valve is stiffened and has a narrowed opening (a condition called stenosis). It does not open properly, which increases strain on the heart because the left ventricle has to pump harder to send blood out to the body. Sometimes the aortic valve also does not close properly, causing it to leak, a condition called aortic regurgitation.
- Atrial Septal Defect (ASD): ASD is a hole in the wall (called the septum) that separates the left atrium and the right atrium.
- Atrioventricular Canal Defect: This defect, also known as endocardial cushion defect, or atrioventricular septal defect, is caused by a poorly formed central area of the heart. Typically, there is a large hole between the upper chambers of the heart (the atria) and often an additional hole between the lower chambers of the heart (the ventricles). Instead of two separate valves allowing flow into the heart (tricuspid on the right and mitral valve on the left), there is one large common valve, which may be quite malformed.
- Coarctation of the Aorta: This is a narrowing of a portion of the aorta and often seriously decreases the blood flow from the heart out to the lower portion of the body.

- Hypoplastic Left Heart Syndrome: When the structures of the left side of the heart (the left ventricle, the mitral valve, and the aortic valve) are underdeveloped, they are unable to pump blood adequately to the entire body. This condition is usually diagnosed within the first few days of life, at which point the infant may be critically ill.
- Patent Ductus Arteriosus (PDA): The ductus arteriosus (DA) is a normal blood vessel in the developing fetus that diverts circulation away from the lungs and sends it directly to the body. The DA usually closes on its own shortly after birth; it is no longer needed once a newborn breathes on his own. If the DA doesn't close, then a condition called patent ductus arteriosus (PDA) results, which can result in too much blood flow to a newborn's lungs. PDA is common in premature babies.
- Pulmonary Atresia: This defect is one where the pulmonic valve does not open at all and may indeed be completely absent. The main blood vessel that runs between the right ventricle and the lungs also may be malformed, and the right ventricle can be abnormally small.
- Pulmonary Stenosis: In pulmonary stenosis, the pulmonic valve is stiffened and has a narrowed opening (a condition called stenosis). It does not open properly, which increases strain on the right side of the heart because the right ventricle has to pump harder to send blood out to the lungs.
- Tetralogy of Fallot (TOF): Tetralogy of Fallot is actually a combination of four heart defects. It in-

cludes pulmonary stenosis, a thickened right ventricle (known as ventricular hypertrophy), a hole between the lower chambers (known as a ventricular septal defect), and an aorta that can receive blood from both the left and right ventricles instead of draining just the left. Because deoxygenated (blue) blood can flow out to the body, children with this defect often appear bluish.

- Total Anomalous Pulmonary Venous Connection: The pulmonary veins normally are the blood vessels that deliver oxygenated blood from the lungs to the left atrium. Sometimes these vessels don't join the left atrium during development. Instead, they deliver blood to the heart by other pathways, which may be narrowed. Pressure builds up in this pathway and in the pulmonary veins, pushing fluid into the lungs, decreasing the amount of oxygenated blood that reaches the body. These infants often have difficulty breathing and appear bluish.
- Transposition of the Great Arteries: In this condition, the pulmonary artery and the aorta (the major blood vessels leaving the heart) are switched so that the aorta arises from the right side of the heart and receives blue blood, which is sent right back out to the body without becoming oxygen-rich. The pulmonary artery rises from the left side of the heart, receives red blood, and sends it back to the lungs again. The result is that babies with this condition often appear very blue and have low oxygen levels in the bloodstream. They usually come to medical attention within the first days of life.

- Tricuspid Atresia: Blood normally flows from the right atrium to the right ventricle through the tricuspid valve. In tricuspid atresia, the valve is replaced by a plate or membrane that does not open. The right ventricle therefore does not receive blood normally and is often small.
- Truncus Arteriosus: In an embryo, the aorta and the pulmonary artery are initially a single vessel. During normal development, that vessel splits to form the two major arteries. If that split does not occur, the child is born with a single common great blood vessel called the truncus arteriosus. There is usually a hole between the ventricles associated with this defect.
- Ventricular Septal Defect (VSD): One of the most common congenital heart defects, VSD is a hole in the wall (septum) between the heart's left and right ventricles. These can occur at different locations and vary in size from very small to very large. Some of the smaller defects may gradually close on their own.

Signs and Symptoms of Heart Defects

Because congenital defects often compromise the heart's ability to pump blood and to deliver oxygen to the tissues of the body, they often produce telltale signs in the child. These may include:

- A bluish tinge or color (cyanosis) to the skin around the mouth or on the lips and tongue

- An increased rate of breathing or difficulty breathing
- Poor appetite or difficulty feeding (which may be associated with color change)
- Failure to thrive (failure to gain weight or weight loss)
- Abnormal heart murmur
- Sweating, especially during feedings
- Diminished strength of the baby's pulse

If the child's doctor thinks that the baby may have a congenital defect, he or she may refer you to a pediatric cardiologist. Some congenital heart defects cause serious symptoms right at birth, requiring newborn intensive care in the hospital and immediate evaluation by a cardiologist. Other defects, like small atrial septal defects, may go undiagnosed until teen or even adult years.

After a complete physical examination, including evaluation of the baby's heart rate and blood pressure, the cardiologist probably will order a chest X-ray to evaluate the size and shape of the heart and to view the lungs.

An electrocardiogram (EKG) is usually done, too. EKGs are performed by placing small pads (called leads) on the child's chest that are wired to a monitor that records and prints out the electrical signals of the heart.

The cardiologist will often order an echocardiogram, which provides detailed images of the heart by using ultrasound. Specialized ultrasound waves can demonstrate blood flow direction and the speed of the flow in various areas of the heart. Echocardiograms are the primary tool for diagnosing congenital heart defects.

A pediatric cardiologist is the doctor most qualified to diagnose a congenital heart defect and provide treatment. Today, there are more treatment options for congenital heart defects than ever before, and most defects are treated successfully.

Persistent Pulmonary Hypertension

Persistent pulmonary hypertension (PPHN) is the presence of blood flow through the lungs and heart seen in the fetus (before the baby is born). While the baby was growing inside the womb, the mother did the breathing for him. Oxygenated blood went from the mother's lungs, through her body, across the placenta, and to the baby. Therefore, the baby did not need to use lungs. Blood was shunted through two channels in the heart called the ductus arteriosus and the foramen ovale and bypassed the baby's lungs. However, after the baby is born, cries, and takes breaths, the pressure in the pulmonary (lung) vessels should decrease; therefore, blood can travel to the lungs to get oxygen. When a baby has PPHN, the pressure in the pulmonary vessels does not decrease, causing blood to shunt the wrong way (away from the lungs), as if the baby were still inside the womb. Therefore, the baby receives unoxygenated blood to his body.

This condition is usually seen in near-term, term, or post-term infants. Symptoms are usually seen in the first twelve hours of life. Several factors can cause PPHN. One cause may be due to a stressful birthing process. The baby may stool, gasp, and swallow meconium (the first few stools, which are thick, sticky, and pasty). The meconium can get into the baby's lungs and cause the baby to have difficulty breathing after birth. Other causes of PPHN may be cold stress, low blood sugar, low calcium, thickening of the blood, or infection.

The symptoms that will be first noticed will be that the baby may begin to breathe faster (tachypnea), and the baby's chest may suck in (retractions) as if he were having a hard time breathing. The baby will probably need to be placed on a breathing machine (ventilator). A nurse will need to give some medication (sedation) to help him rest. You may see a bluish discoloration of the skin (cyanosis) because of decreased oxygen. The baby's blood pressure may also be low. The main goal is to get oxygenated blood to the rest of the baby's body. The ventilator and medications will do this. The baby may need to be on a special medication to increase his blood pressure (vasopressor). The baby will have several lines and intravenous accesses to measure and monitor his condition. PPHN is a very serious condition. Some babies show long-term developmental problems; therefore, the baby's development should be closely evaluated.

Endocrine

Diabetes Insipidus

Diabetes insipidus is a disorder in which there is an abnormal increase in urine output, fluid intake, and often thirst. It causes symptoms such as urinary frequency, nocturia (frequent awakening at night to urinate) or enuresis (involuntary urination during sleep or bedwetting). Urine output is increased because it is not concentrated normally. Consequently, instead of being a yellow color, the urine is pale, colorless, or watery in appearance, and the measured concentration (osmolality or specific gravity) is low.

Diabetes insipidus is not the same as diabetes mellitus (sugar diabetes). Diabetes insipidus resembles diabetes mellitus because the symptoms of both diseases are increased urination and thirst. However, in every other respect, including the causes and treatment of the disorders, the diseases are completely unrelated. Sometimes diabetes insipidus is referred to as water diabetes to distinguish it from the more common diabetes mellitus or sugar diabetes.

Diabetes insipidus is divided into four types, each of which has a different cause and must be treated differently. The most common type of DI is caused by a lack of vasopressin, a hormone that normally acts upon the kidney to reduce urine output by increasing the concentration of the urine. This type of DI is usually due to the destruction of the back or posterior part of the pituitary gland where vasopressin is normally produced. It is commonly called pituitary DI. It is also known as central or neurogenci DI.

Diabetes Mellitus

Diabetes is a disease that affects how the body uses glucose, the main type of sugar in the blood. Glucose comes from the foods we eat and is the major source of energy needed to fuel the body's functions.

After you eat a meal, your body breaks down the foods you eat into glucose and other nutrients, which are then absorbed into the bloodstream from the gastrointestinal tract. The glucose level in the blood rises after a meal and triggers the pancreas to make the hormone insulin and release it into the bloodstream. But in people with diabetes, the body either can't make or can't respond to insulin properly.

Insulin works like a key that opens the doors to cells and allows the glucose in. Without insulin, glucose can't get into the cells and so it stays in the bloodstream. As a result, the level of sugar in the blood remains higher than normal. High blood sugar levels are a problem because they can cause a number of health problems.

There are two major types of diabetes: type 1 and type 2. Both type 1 and type 2 diabetes cause blood sugar levels to become higher than normal. However, they cause it in different ways.

Type 1 diabetes (formerly called insulin-dependent diabetes or juvenile diabetes) results when the pancreas loses its ability to make the hormone insulin. In type 1 diabetes, the person's own immune system attacks and destroys the cells in the pancreas that produce insulin. Once those cells are destroyed, they won't ever make insulin again.

Type 1 diabetes can't be prevented, and there is no practical way to predict who will get it. There is nothing that either a parent or the child did to cause the disease. Once a person has type 1 diabetes, it does not go away and requires lifelong treatment. Children and teens with type

1 diabetes depend on daily insulin injections or an insulin pump to control their blood glucose levels.

Type 2 diabetes (formerly called noninsulin-dependent diabetes or adult-onset diabetes) is different from type 1 diabetes. Type 2 diabetes results from the body's inability to respond to insulin normally. Unlike people with type 1 diabetes, most people with type 2 diabetes can still produce insulin but not enough to meet their body's needs.

Signs and Symptoms of Type 1 Diabetes

A person can have diabetes without knowing it because the symptoms aren't always obvious, and they can take a long time to develop. Type 1 diabetes may come on gradually or suddenly.

Parents of a child (or foster parent with a child under your care) with typical symptoms of type 1 diabetes may notice that their child:

- Urinates frequently: The kidneys respond to high levels of glucose in the bloodstream by flushing out the extra glucose in urine. A child with diabetes needs to urinate more frequently and in larger volumes and is abnormally thirsty. Because the child is losing so much fluid from peeing so much, he or she becomes very thirsty to help avoid becoming dehydrated. A child who has developed diabetes drinks a lot in an attempt to keep the level of body water normal.
- Loses weight: (or fails to gain weight as he or she grows) in spite of a good appetite. Kids and

teens that develop type 1 diabetes may have an increased appetite but often lose weight. This is because the body breaks down muscle and stored fat in an attempt to provide fuel to the hungry cells.

- Often feels tired: because the body can't use glucose for energy properly.

But in some cases, other symptoms may be the signal that something is wrong. Sometimes the first sign of diabetes is bedwetting in a child who has been dry at night. The possibility of diabetes should also be suspected if a vaginal yeast infection (also called a Candida infection) occurs in a girl who hasn't started puberty yet.

If these early symptoms of diabetes aren't recognized and treatment isn't started, chemicals called ketones can build up in the child's blood and cause stomach pain, nausea, vomiting, fruity-smelling breath, breathing problems, and even loss of consciousness. Sometimes these symptoms are mistaken for the flu or appendicitis. Doctors call this serious condition diabetic ketoacidosis, or DKA.

In addition to short-term problems like those listed above, diabetes can also cause long-term complications in some people, including heart disease, stroke, vision impairment, and kidney damage. Diabetes can also cause other problems throughout the body in the blood vessels, nerves, and gums. These problems don't usually show up in kids or teens with type 1 diabetes who have had the disease for only a few years. However, these health problems can occur in adulthood in some people with diabetes particularly if they haven't managed or controlled their diabetes properly.

Proper treatment can stop or control these diabetes symptoms and reduce the risk of long-term problems. Doctors can say for sure if a person has diabetes by testing blood samples for glucose. If the diagnosis of diabetes is suspected or confirmed, the doctor will refer your child to a pediatric endocrinologist, a doctor who specializes in the diagnosis and treatment of children with diseases of the endocrine system such as diabetes and growth disorders.

Panhypopituitarism

Hypopituitarism refers to a deficiency of one or more of the hormones secreted by the anterior pituitary gland. Panhypopituitarism refers to an absence of all hormones released by the pituitary gland. Pituitary insufficiency in the adult is most commonly caused by a nonfunctioning tumor or surgical removal or irradiation of the pituitary gland.

The lack of pituitary hormones results in a reduction in the hormones released by the target glands (i.e., thyroid, adrenals, and gonads). When hypo- or pan-hypopituitarism results from inherent disease or irradiation, symptoms develop gradually. After surgery, symptoms of adrenal sufficiency can develop within days and hypothyroidism after only a month.

In panhypopituitarism, facial and body hair decrease and reproductive organs and muscle tissue shrivel. There can be loss of libido, impotency, amenorrhea, and infertility. Hypoglycemia may occur due to a deficiency of growth hormone. There is also a loss of normal skin pigmentation, which can become pale and waxy in appearance. Wrinkles may develop around the eyes and mouth, making the person appear older than normal. When pituitary deficiency is severe, there is extreme weight loss, emaciation with eventual coma, and if untreated, death.

Because pituitary hormones are destroyed in the gastrointestinal tract, treatment of hypopituitarism involves replacement of the deficient hormones of the target organs. Additionally, within the last five years, the FDA approved growth hormone for treatment in those with panhypopituitarism. Growth hormone is self-administered by injection, subcutaneously, on a daily basis.

Gastrointestinal

Gastroesophageal Reflux

Gastroesophageal reflux disease (GE reflux or GERD) is the backward flow of stomach contents into the esophagus (food pipe). It is caused when the muscle at the entrance to the stomach is immature and allows the food to move back up into the esophagus and throat.

Apnea (no breathing) and bradycardia (low heart rate), difficulty feeding or refusing to eat, choking episodes, lots of spitting, coughing spells, or wheezing could all be symptoms of gastro-esophageal reflux.

Gastroesophageal reflux can be diagnosed from the symptoms that you report to the doctor and by utilizing the following tests:

- Upper GI: the baby is fed a harmless dye, and X-rays are taken as the dye goes through the stomach and intestines
- PH Probe: a tiny probe is put in the baby's esophagus. If stomach contents are moving back up into the esophagus, the probe will show too much acid there.

The baby will be first treated by being placed on some medicines. The baby's feedings may be thickened with rice cereal. The baby will also be placed on reflux precautions to help prevent aspiration (breathing in stomach contents into the lungs). A small number of infants will require surgery.

These are simple things that you can do to make it less likely that the baby will have problems:

- The baby should sleep in a crib with the mattress elevated to a forty-five-degree angle. This can be done by placing a wedge, using folded blankets or towels, under the head of the mattress.
- Do not lay the baby flat on his or her back when feeding and immediately after feeding. Keep the baby in a head-up position for twenty minutes after feeding.
- Schedule diaper changes, baths, dressing, and active playing to occur before feedings.
- Avoid activities such as tickling, bouncing, or excessive rocking during or immediately after feeding, that cause spitting up.

Many infants outgrow GE reflux by ten to twelve months of age. The absence of symptoms does not guarantee that the infant has outgrown the disease.

Nissen fundoplication surgery is the final option for controlling very severe gastroesophageal reflux disease. Because of the possible complications that can accompany this surgery, it is typically done as a last resort. It is by no means a cure for GERD and is only performed when severe symptoms and complications persist. It involves wrapping the upper portion of the stomach (fundus) around the lower portion of the esophagus.

Gastroschisis

Gastroschisis is a defect that occurs when the abdominal wall fails to close properly during fetal development, allowing the intestines to protrude through the abdominal wall. Gastroschisis is usually discovered when the mother's alpha-fetoprotein (AFP) blood levels become elevated during the second trimester. The problem may also be detected during a routine fetal ultrasound.

Gastroschisis occurs in approximately one in five thousand births. It does not appear to run in families, and there is no increased risk of recurrence in future pregnancies.

Unfortunately, we do not know the exact cause of gastroschisis. However, it is often associated with younger mothers (under twenty years of age) and is unrelated to anything the mother ate or did before or during her pregnancy. Gastroschisis usually occurs as an isolated defect and is not typically seen in conjunction with other health problems.

During the third trimester, the baby is at risk for gastroschisis-related complications such as bowel dilatation (stretching), decreased fetal growth rate, oligohydramnios (low volume of amniotic fluid, indicating reduced fetal kidney function), and in only very rare cases, death. For this reason, mothers and babies are closely monitored with ultrasound and fetal non-stress testing.

The fetal non-stress test monitors the baby's heart function. It records the heart rate of the fetus while he or she is moving. If the heart is functioning properly, the fetal heart rate should increase in response to movement.

The condition of the fetus is carefully monitored to determine the best time for delivery. After delivery, surgical correction of gastroschisis involves the return of any exposed bowel to the abdominal cavity and subsequent closure of the abdominal wall. This can be accomplished in one of two ways:

1. Primary gastroschisis repair: The baby undergoes surgical repair immediately after birth. The bowel is returned to the abdominal cavity, and the abdominal wall is closed during one procedure. This is the preferred method of repair because it is associated with a reduced risk of infection and fluid loss.
2. Staged gastroschisis repair: Prolonged exposure to irritating amniotic fluid or trauma during birth may inflame or stretch the bowel. If so, the bowel is covered by a sheet of protective material and gradually returns to the abdominal cavity by gravity. Then the abdomen is closed

surgically. The method chosen depends upon the condition of the bowel after birth.

Although the abdomen is closed after the gastroschisis repair, it takes time for the intestines to recover from gastroschisis. For this reason, first feedings are provided intravenously. Once bowel function returns, as evidenced by the passing of a bowel movement, feedings via a nasogastric (NG) tube are slowly initiated while IV feeds continue. NG feeds are slowly increased, as tolerated, and oral feeding is introduced. This is a gradual process, and infants who have undergone gastroschisis repair might experience occasional setbacks, including need for bowel rest or additional surgery.

When the infant who has undergone gastroschisis repair can tolerate full feedings via a combination of oral and NG feeds with adequate weight gain, he or she is getting ready to go home. Prior to discharge, teaching of special feeding techniques or other specialized care will be provided to the foster parents by the nursing staff.

The length of stay in the hospital after gastroschisis repair varies depending on the above outlined factors. After discharge from the hospital, the infant will be closely monitored by his or her pediatrician or with other specialists as needed.

Hirschsprung's Disease

Hirschsprung's disease occurs when some of the nerve cells that are normally present in the intestine do not form properly while a baby is developing during pregnancy. As food is digested, muscles move food forward through the intestines in a movement called peristalsis. When we eat, nerve cells that are present in the wall of the intestines receive signals from the brain telling the intestinal muscles to move food forward.

In children with Hirschsprung's disease, a lack of nerve cells in part of the intestine interrupts the signal from the brain and prevents peristalsis in that segment of the intestine. Because stool cannot move forward normally, the intestine can become partially or completely obstructed (blocked) and begins to expand to a larger than normal size.

The problems a child will experience with Hirschsprung's disease depend on how much of the intestine has normal nerve cells present. Seventy percent of babies with Hirschsprung's disease are missing nerve cells in only the last one to two feet of the large intestine.

Between the fifth and twelfth weeks of pregnancy, while the fetus is growing and developing, nerve cells form in the digestive tract, beginning in the mouth and finishing in the anus. For unknown reasons, the nerve cells do not grow past a certain point in the intestine in babies with Hirschsprung's disease.

Scientists are not sure why the intestinal nerve cells do not form completely. Nothing has been shown to cause this problem, including medications a mother takes while pregnant or what a mother eats during pregnancy.

Hirschsprung's disease occurs five times more frequently in males than in females. Children with Down syndrome have a higher risk of having Hirschsprung's disease.

There is possibly a genetic, or inherited, cause for

Hirschsprung's disease. If a family has a child with Hirschsprung's disease, there is a 3 to 12 percent chance that another baby they have will also have the disease. Also, there is an increased chance that a couple will have a child with Hirschsprung's disease if one of the parents has the disease. The chances are higher if the mother is the parent with Hirschsprung's disease.

In a patient with Hirschsprung's disease, a segment of the intestine lacks normal nerve cells. Digested food and stool cannot move forward through that portion of the digestive tract. The intestine becomes blocked with stool, and the baby will be constipated or unable to have normal bowel movements.

The obstruction (blockage) causes pressure on the inside of the intestine, causing part of the intestinal wall to wear thin. Eventually, a bacterial infection can develop in the digestive tract, causing serious problems. Eighty percent of children with Hirschsprung's disease show symptoms in the first six weeks of life. Children who only have a short segment of intestine that lacks normal nerve cells may not show symptoms for several months or years. The following are the most common symptoms of Hirschsprung's disease. However, each individual may experience symptoms differently. Symptoms may include:

- Not having a bowel movement in the first forty-eight hours of life
- Gradual bloating of the abdomen
- Gradual onset of vomiting
- Fever

Children who do not have early symptoms may also present the following:

- Constipation that becomes worse with time
- Gradual bloating of the abdomen
- Gradual onset of vomiting
- Fever
- Loss of appetite
- Delayed growth
- Passing small, watery stools

Symptoms of Hirschsprung's disease may resemble other conditions or medical problems. It can be diagnosed from physical exam, medical history, and tests that may include:

- Abdominal X-ray: a diagnostic test that may show a lack of stool in the large intestine or near the anus and dilated segments of the large and small intestine
- Barium enema: a procedure performed to examine the large intestine for abnormalities. Fluid called barium (a metallic, chemical, chalky, liquid used to coat the inside of organs so that they will show up on an X-ray) is given into the rectum as an enema. An X-ray of the abdomen shows strictures (narrowed areas), obstructions (blockages), and dilated intestine above the obstruction.
- Anorectal manometry: a test that measures nerve reflexes that are missing in Hirschsprung's disease

- Biopsy of the rectum or large intestine: a test that takes a sample of the cells in the rectum or large intestine and then looks for nerve cells under a microscope

Specific treatment for Hirschsprung's disease will be determined by the child's physician based on the following:

- The extent of the problem
- The child's age, overall health, and medical history
- The child's tolerance for specific medications, procedures, or therapies
- Expectations for the course of the disorder
- The opinion of the physicians involved in the child's care

An operation is usually necessary to deal with intestinal obstruction caused by Hirschsprung's disease. The surgeon removes the portion of the rectum and intestine that lacks normal nerve cells. A colostomy is done so stool can leave the body. With a colostomy, the upper end of the intestine is brought through an opening in the abdomen known as a stoma. Stool will pass through the opening and then into a collection bag. The colostomy may be temporary or permanent depending on the amount of intestine that is needs to be removed. After a healing period, many children can have the intestine surgically reconnected above to the anal opening and have the colostomy closed.

Children who have a large section of intestine removed may have long-term problems. When a large portion of the intestine is removed, the digestive process can be affected. Nutrients and fluids are absorbed from food in the small intestine. Removing a large segment of the intestine can prevent a child from getting adequate nutrients and fluids. Children can have problems with improper digestion, slow growth, and infection.

Necrotizing Enterocolitis

Necrotizing means causing death to tissue, entero refers to the small intestine, colo refers to the large intestine, and -itis is inflammation. Necrotizing enterocolitis is an inflammation that could cause destruction of part of the bowel. NEC may involve only the innermost lining or the entire thickness of the bowel and variable amounts of the bowel.

Premature infants get NEC because they have immature and fragile bowels. They are sensitive to changes in blood flow and to infection. We often do not know why an individual baby develops NEC. NEC usually occurs when babies are three to twelve days old but may develop when they are several weeks old. It usually begins a few days after feedings are started. However, babies fed fresh breast milk get NEC less often.

NEC is very serious because the baby can lose some of their bowel from it. For this reason, doctors may start treatment on simply the suspicion that the baby might be developing symptoms of NEC. This suspicion is sometimes referred to as "rule out NEC," "possible NEC," or a "NEC scare."

Symptoms may be mild or severe. The baby may show any or all of the following:

- General signs of being sick: less active, more apnea, increased respiratory problems, difficulty keeping his or her body temperature normal
- Poor tolerance to feedings, vomiting, or having milk sit in the stomach (called aspirates or residuals); these residuals may be greenish in color
- Increased size of the abdomen
- Redness or abnormal color to the abdomen
- Blood in the stool

If the baby's doctor thinks that he or she might be developing NEC, any or all of the following might be done:

- All regular feedings stopped. This is called NPO. The baby will have an IV started so he or she can be fed by vein.
- A tube placed into the stomach either from the mouth or nose and hooked to a suction machine. The tube removes air and fluids from the baby's stomach and intestine.
- The abdomen size measured with a tape measure and watched carefully.
- X-rays of the abdomen.

- A sample of the blood sent to the laboratory to see if it contains bacteria.
- Antibiotics started.
- More frequent blood tests to look for signs of infection and imbalances in the body's chemistry.
- Oxygen started or increased; the baby may have to go on a ventilator.

If part of the baby's intestine dies and only the innermost lining of bowel dies, the body can slowly regrow it. If the entire thickness of a piece of the bowel dies, the baby will need surgery to remove that piece of the bowel. The end of the bowel above the removed segment may be brought to the surface of the skin (called ostomy). At some later time, after the baby has recovered and grown much bigger, the two ends of the bowel can be sewn back together again.

Most babies who recover from NEC do not have further problems, but future problems are possible. These include scarring and narrowing of the bowel causing obstruction or blockage of the bowel and malabsorption or the inability of the bowel to absorb nutrients normally.

Genetic Disorders

Cystic Fibrosis

Cystic fibrosis (CF) is an inherited disease that causes the body to produce mucus that's extremely thick and sticky. The mucus in people with CF is thicker than normal because CF affects cells in the epithelium the layer of cells that lines the passages in the body's organs. In a person who does not have CF, the epithelial cells produce thin, watery mucus that acts like a lubricant and helps protect the body's tissues. In a person with CF, however, the thicker mucus doesn't move as easily. This thick, sticky mucus clogs passages in many of the body's organs and infection sets in.

The two organs that are most affected are the lungs and pancreas, where the thick mucus causes breathing and digestive problems. The thicker mucus has trouble moving out of the lungs, so bacteria can remain and cause infections. The thick mucus can also be found in the pancreas, an organ that produces proteins called enzymes that flow into the intestine to support the body's digestion process. Because the mucus can block the path between the pancreas and the intestines, people with CF have trouble digesting food and getting the vitamins and nutrients they need from it. CF can also affect the liver, the sweat glands, and the reproductive organs.

Cystic fibrosis is an inherited disease caused by mutations (changes) in a gene on chromosome 7, one of the twenty-three pairs of chromosomes that children inherit from their parents. Cystic fibrosis occurs because of mutations in the gene that makes a protein called CFTR (cystic fibrosis transmembrane regulator). A person with CF produces abnormal CFTR protein or no CFTR protein at all, which causes the body to make thick, sticky mucus instead of the thin, watery kind.

People who are born with CF have two copies of the CF gene. In almost all people born with CF, one gene is received from each parent. This means that the parents of kids with CF are usually both CF carriers, that is, they have one normal and one defective gene, but the parents may not have CF themselves because their normal gene is able to take over and make the necessary CFTR protein. Each child born to parents who are both CF carriers has a one in four chance of having the disease. Doctors can also perform tests during pregnancy so prospective parents can find out more about the chances that their child will have CF. However, these tests also won't always detect a CF gene.

Doctors diagnose most kids with CF by the time they are three years old, but if someone has a milder form of the disease, it may not be diagnosed until that person reaches the teen years. Babies are usually tested if they are born with an intestinal blockage called meconium ileus, which is more common in CF infants.

Other symptoms include:

- Frequent lung infections or pneumonia
- Persistent wheezing
- Persistent cough with thick mucus
- Bulky, light-colored, foul-smelling bowel movements or diarrhea (because food isn't being digested properly)
- Failure to gain weight, even though the child eats normal amounts
- Very salty sweat
- Poor height growth

- Nasal polyps (small growths of tissue inside the nose)
- Frequent sinus infections
- Fatigue

People with CF get frequent lung infections that can damage their lungs over time and require strong antibiotics, along with stays in the hospital. They may have trouble growing or gaining weight because of digestive problems. Adults with CF may also develop other illnesses, such as osteoporosis. The ends of the toes and fingers may become rounded and enlarged, a condition that's called clubbing.

If doctors suspect that a person has CF, they will order a sweat test. In this test, the doctor or technician uses a chemical and a very mild electrical current to cause sweating on an area of skin, usually on a person's forearm (this test doesn't hurt). The doctor or technician collects a large amount of sweat in a pad and then analyzes it. If the test results show a high level of chloride (a chemical in salt), there's a possibility the person has CF.

Doctors and people with CF can do several things to slow the progression of the disease and fight its complications. To loosen mucus, people with CF exercise regularly and may use inhalers or nebulizers that help deliver medication to the lungs.

Coughing helps people with CF clear the mucus from their lungs. They may also take antibiotics to prevent or fight lung infections. Chest physical therapy may also be an important part of a person's CF treatment routine.

After lying down in a position that helps drain mucus from the lungs, the person has a helper, such as a parent, gently bang on his or her chest or back to loosen the mucus. A newer device called a therapy vest that shakes the chest allows teens to be more independent by doing their therapy on their own.

For digestive problems, a person with CF can take enzymes by mouth in order to help digest food and get nutrients from it. A doctor may also prescribe vitamin supplements and a high-calorie diet. Right now, there is no cure for CF. Even if symptoms are mild at first, they get steadily worse over time.

Fragile X Syndrome

Fragile X syndrome is a chromosomal birth defect. This syndrome primarily affects males (one in 1,500). Although one in one thousand females is a carrier, only one in three shows outward signs of having the defect, including intellectual impairment. The range of retardation varies from mild to severe.

Symptoms: The physical characteristics of Fragile X syndrome may include large ears, an elongated face, poor muscle tone, flat feet, large testicles, overcrowded teeth, cleft palate, heart problems, and autisticlike tendencies. Affected children may also suffer seizures.

However, many children with Fragile X syndrome appear to be physically normal at birth, so a diagnosis may not be made until the ages of eighteen months and two years. At that time, a lack of language development coupled with other developmental delays usually prompts testing.

Treatment: As with Down syndrome, children with Fragile X syndrome can be expected to do most things that any young child can do, although they also generally learn these things later than unaffected children. And, as with most of these birth defects, early intervention programs begun in infancy can help maximize the child's development.

Hemophilia

Hemophilia is a disease that prevents blood from clotting properly, so a person who has it bleeds more than someone without hemophilia does. It's a genetic disorder, which means it's the result of a change in genes that was either inherited (passed on from parent to child) or occurred during development in the womb. Hemo means blood and philia means a tendency toward. A person who has hemophilia has a tendency to bleed excessively. Hemophilia affects mostly boys, although it's very rare. The disease can affect people of any race or nationality.

When most people get a cut, the body naturally protects itself. Sticky cells in the blood called platelets go to where the bleeding is and plug up the hole. This is the first step in the clotting process. When the platelets plug the hole, they release chemicals that attract more sticky platelets and also activate various proteins in the blood known as clotting factors. These proteins mix with the platelets to form fibers, and these fibers make the clot stronger and stop the bleeding.

Our bodies have twelve clotting factors that work together in this process (numbered using Roman numerals from I through XII). Having too little of factors VIII (8) and IX (9) is what causes hemophilia. A person with hemophilia will only lack one factor, either factor VIII or factor IX but not both.

There are two major kinds of hemophilia. About 80 percent of cases are hemophilia A, which is a factor VIII deficiency. Hemophilia B is when factor IX is lacking.

Hemophilia is classified as mild, moderate, or severe based on the amount of the clotting factor in the person's blood. If someone produces only 1 percent or less of the affected factor, the case is called severe. Someone that produces 2 percent to 5 percent has a moderate case, and someone that produces 6 percent to 50 percent of the affected factor level is considered to have a mild case of hemophilia. In general, a person with milder hemophilia may only bleed excessively once in a while, whereas severe hemophilia puts someone at risk for having bleeding problems much more often.

Most people with hemophilia discover they have the condition when they are babies or young kids. Sometimes the disease is so mild that it may not be known until he has minor surgery, like getting his tonsils or appendix out, and it's found in blood tests that doctors perform before surgery.

Men and women each have twenty-three pairs of chromosomes. Women have two X chromosomes; men have one X and one Y chromosome. Hemophilia is an X-linked genetic disorder, which means that it's passed from mother to son on the X chromosome. If the mother carries the gene for hemophilia on one of her X chromosomes, each of her sons will have a 50 percent chance of having hemophilia.

Although girls rarely develop the symptoms of hemophilia itself, they can be carriers of the disease. For a girl to get hemophilia, she would have to receive the disease on the chromosome she receives from her father, who would have hemophilia, as well as from the X chromosome of her mother, who would be a carrier. Although this is not impossible, it is highly unlikely.

Symptoms of hemophilia include:

- Bruises that are unusual in location or number
- Nosebleeds that won't or are difficult to stop
- Excessive bleeding from biting a lip or having a tooth pulled
- Painful or swollen joints
- Blood in the urine

Doctors diagnose hemophilia by performing blood tests. Although the disease can't be cured (except by a liver transplant), it can be managed.

A cut or minor wound is usually no big deal for a person with hemophilia, just as it isn't for someone without the disease. However, internal bleeding can be serious. When bleeding occurs in the joints, muscles, or internal body organs, treatment is necessary. Patients with more serious cases of hemophilia often get regular shots of the factor that they're missing—known as clotting factor replacement therapy—to prevent bleeding episodes. The clotting factors are transfused to the person through an IV to his vein and can be given in the hospital, at the doctor's office, or at home. People with moderate or mild cases of hemophilia usually don't need these shots unless they have a serious injury or require surgery.

If you have an infant under your care that has hemophilia, you will probably get used to working with a medical team of hematologists (doctors who specialize in blood disorders), nurses, and social workers.

The medical team can help you learn to recognize bleeding internally. This is important to know because when the infant or child begins to bleed internally, you need to infuse (replace) the missing clotting factor right away to make the bleeding stop. Putting off doing so can cause damage to the joints.

If you will be injecting the clotting factors at home, the treatment team will teach you how to mix the clotting factor and inject it into a vein. If the infant or child under your care has bleeds fairly often, though, the doctor might consider having infusion of the clotting factor regularly to prevent bleeds from happening in the first place. If that's the case, the patient might get a small tube called a porta-cath, or port, implanted into his or her chest. That way no one will have to worry about finding a vein and there's no pain when the infusion is done.

Pierre Robin Sequence

Pierre Robin sequence describes the sequence of events that happen while the mother is pregnant that cause the baby to develop as follows.

When mom is seven to eleven weeks pregnant (one to three months), something happens to cause the baby's jaw to form smaller than usual. This, in turn, causes the tongue to be placed in an abnormal position and makes the roof of the mouth to be high and more toward the back than it should be. Then this causes the roof of the mouth not to close like it should, resulting in a cleft palate and a narrow breathing tube. This can result in the baby's having trouble breathing because of the narrow breathing tube and the tongue being in the way.

The baby will be examined by many doctors, which may include an ear, nose, and throat specialist, a doctor specializing in surgical repair of the mouth.

The largest percentages of these babies do very well and have minimal breathing problems. However, there are a small number of babies with significant breathing problems requiring assistance with breathing. Breathing difficulty can be managed with something as simple as positioning, or may require surgery since the blood travels to all parts of the body. The bacteria or germs may cause intervention (tracheostomy). Frequently, these babies have breathing problems due to their cleft palate and large tongue. Often, this can be managed by using a special nipple. The repair of the cleft palate will be done at a later date, usually around one year of age.

Treacher Collins Syndrome

Treacher Collins syndrome is a condition that affects the development of bones and other tissues in the face. Treacher Collins syndrome is believed to be caused by a change in the gene on chromosome 5, which affects facial development. About 40 percent of the time, one parent has the Treacher Collins syndrome gene. Geneticists can now determine whether the Treacher Collins gene is a new mutation or one that has been passed on.

The signs and symptoms of this disorder vary greatly, ranging from almost unnoticeable to severe. Most affected individuals have underdeveloped facial bones, particularly the cheekbones, and a very small jaw and chin (micrognathia). Some people with this condition are also born with an opening in the roof of the mouth called a cleft palate. In severe cases, underdevelopment of the facial bones may restrict an affected infant's airway, causing potentially life-threatening respiratory problems. This condition is also characterized by absent, small, or unusually formed ears. Defects in the middle ear (which contains three small bones that transmit sound) cause hearing loss in about half of cases.

Most children with Treacher Collins have normal development and intelligence; however, it is important that there be early hearing tests. Most children with Treacher Collins syndrome benefit from early intervention speech and language programs.

Depending on the severity of the Treacher Collins, the child may need some or all of the following procedures:

- A conductive hearing aid
- Correction of the cleft palate
- Repair of the sidewall and floor of the eye socket
- Repair of the cheekbones
- Repair of the eyelid notches
- Correction of the undeveloped jaw and chin
- Surgery to correct the beaklike nose
- Reconstruction of the ears

Velo-Cardio-Facial Syndrome

Velo-Cardio-Facial syndrome (VCFS), also known as 22q11.2 deletion syndrome, Shprintzen syndrome and DiGeorge sequence, is caused by the deletion of a small segment of the long arm of chromosome 22 (specified as 22q11.2 deletion) and is one of the most common genetic disorders in humans. Velo-Cardio-Facial syndrome is characterized by cleft palate, heart abnormalities, learning disabilities, and over 180 other clinical findings.

VCFS is a multiple anomaly syndrome caused by a submicroscopic deletion of genetic material from the long arm of chromosome 22. This region contains forty genes and the absence of these genes from one copy of chromosome 22 can cause a wide array of problems. In fact, over 180 disorders might occur in VCFS, and they cover nearly every organ system in the body, with broad reaching effects on development and behavior, including speech, language, personality, mood, learning, attention, and temperament.

Some of the major problems include speech disorders,

heart anomalies, feeding problems, ADD or ADHD, psychiatric illness, immune disorders, and cleft palate, to name just a few. Although genetic testing is available for VCFS, it usually is diagnosed by physical examination at birth. VCFS can exhibit different characteristics in different children, and therefore it is important that a knowledgeable team of specialists evaluate a child so that nothing is overlooked.

Shortly after birth, the child should be seen at the craniofacial center; they will make sure he or she is able to adequately feed and breathe, since swallowing problems are common in babies with VCFS. Within the first two months of life, the infant should be seen for a full craniofacial team evaluation so that appropriate referrals can be made to treat the child's unique needs. Heart defects should be diagnosed and treated by an experienced pediatric cardiologist. Immune deficiencies should be diagnosed and treated by an experienced pediatric endocrinologist.

Some children with VCFS experience speech difficulties even when the palate looks normal. In addition, orthodontic treatment may be necessary.

If there is evidence of developmental delay, the child should be referred to an infant stimulation program to receive thorough developmental testing and appropriate interventions. A child with VCFS may encounter social and emotional challenges unique to this condition.

Infections

HIV and AIDS

HIV (human immunodeficiency virus) is a virus that attacks the immune system (the body's defense against infection). HIV uses healthy white blood cells to replicate itself, breaking down the immune system and leaving the body more susceptible to illness. Without treatment, most people infected with HIV become less able to fight off germs that we are exposed to every day. Someone who has HIV is called HIV positive.

AIDS (acquired immune deficiency syndrome) is a late stage of HIV infection. An HIV-positive person is diagnosed with AIDS when his or her immune system is so weakened that it is no longer able to fight off illness. People with immune deficiency are much more vulnerable to infections such as pneumonia and various forms of cancer. These diseases are called opportunistic infections because they take advantage of the weakened immune system. Ultimately, people do not die from AIDS itself; they die from one or more of these opportunistic infections. It is believed that all people who become HIV positive will eventually have AIDS.

There is no known cure or vaccine for AIDS. While antiviral medications and healthy behavior can improve the quality and length of life for some people living with AIDS, these treatments do not work for everyone and may cause harmful side effects. It can take several years before HIV breaks down a person's immune system and causes AIDS, and people may show few symptoms for several years after they are infected. People who appear perfectly healthy may not know they have the virus and can pass it on to others. The only way to know if a child has HIV is to get tested.

HIV is transmitted from person to person through the exchange of bodily fluids. While the HIV virus can be found in all bodily fluids of an infected person, only these fluids contain a high enough concentration of HIV to transmit the virus:

- Blood
- Semen (including pre-cum)
- Vaginal secretions
- Breast milk

Modes of Transmission:

- Sexual: unprotected anal, vaginal, or oral sex
- Sharing needles: IV, drug use, tattooing, piercing
- Maternal-Child: before, during, and after birth, including breastfeeding
- Blood transfusion before 1985
- Donor products
- Job injury
- Sharing of sex toys

HIV has not been proven transmittable by saliva, urine, feces, sweat, tears, vomit, or mucus.

HIV is not transmitted through casual contact including hugging, kissing, using public toilets, sharing eating utensils, pools, or coughing.

The most common ways that people put themselves at risk for HIV infection are engaging in unprotected oral, anal, or vaginal sex, sharing unclean drug paraphernalia, like syringes and cookers, or sharing unclean needles used for tattoos and body piercing with a person who is HIV positive or unaware of his or her HIV status.

Children with AIDS may get the same opportunistic infections as adults with the disease. In addition, they also may have severe forms of the typically common childhood bacterial infections, such as conjunctivitis (pink eye), ear infections, and tonsillitis. Babies born to mothers infected with HIV may or may not be infected with the virus, but all carry their mothers' antibodies to HIV for several months. If these babies lack symptoms, health care providers cannot make a definitive diagnosis of HIV infection using standard antibody tests. Instead, they are using new technologies to detect HIV and more accurately determine HIV infection in infants between ages three months and fifteen months. Researchers are evaluating a number of blood tests to determine which ones are best for diagnosing HIV infection in babies younger than three months.

Diarrhea

Diarrhea (loose, watery bowel movements) is a common problem in young children. Diarrhea may be due to a serious illness, but usually it is only the result of a minor infection. The danger of a child having diarrhea is becoming dehydrated. The smaller the child (decreased body weight), the faster he or she can become dehydrated. Increasing the amount of liquid the child drinks can usually prevent dehydration. You may have to offer small sips of fluids every thirty minutes. It is okay to cut down on the solid foods for twenty-four to forty-eight hours so that an increased amount of fluids can be taken in.

Call the child's doctor if any of the following occurs:

- If the child suddenly develops a high fever 101 degrees Fahrenheit axillary
- If stomach pain becomes severe or is more than occasional cramps
- If the diarrhea becomes bloody (more than a streak of blood)
- If the diarrhea becomes more frequent or is more severe
- If the child becomes dehydrated (see signs of dehydration below)
- If there is no improvement in twenty-four to forty-eight hours

Signs of dehydration:

- Infant's soft spot (fontanelle) on top of his head is sunken
- Child has not urinated for six hours
- There are no tears when he cries
- Child's mouth becomes dry or sticky to touch

- Child's eyes are sunken and the skin around the eyes is dark
- Child is less active than usual or is difficult to waken up.

Do not use stool binders or anti-diarrhea medicines for children under six years of age unless your doctor specifically directs it for the child. These medicines can be very dangerous if they are not used properly. When a germ that is contagious causes diarrhea, you can help to protect other family members best by using good hand-washing techniques.

Endocarditis

The inside of the heart contains four chambers and four valves lined by a thin membrane called the endocardium. Endocarditis is an infection of this inner lining. Endocarditis typically occurs when bacteria or other germs from another part of the body, such as the mouth, spread through the bloodstream and attach to damaged areas in the heart. Left untreated, endocarditis can damage or destroy the heart valves. Endocarditis can be life threatening.

Endocarditis is uncommon in people with healthy hearts. People at greatest risk of endocarditis have a damaged heart valve, an artificial heart valve, or other heart defects. Endocarditis may develop slowly or suddenly, depending on what's causing the infection and whether the patient has any underlying heart abnormalities.

Signs and symptoms of endocarditis may include:

- Fever
- Chills
- A new or changed heart murmur
- Fatigue
- Aching joints and muscles
- Night sweats
- Shortness of breath
- Paleness
- Persistent cough
- Swelling in feet, legs, or abdomen
- Unexplained weight loss
- Blood in urine
- Tenderness in spleen, an infection-fighting abdominal organ on your left side, just below your ribcage

Sometimes endocarditis causes red, tender spots under the skin of the fingers. These are known as Osler's nodes. The patient may notice tiny purple or red spots known as petechiae on other areas of the skin. Similar spots may appear in the whites of the eyes or inside the mouth.

Endocarditis occurs when germs enter the bloodstream, travel to the heart, and attach to abnormal heart valves or damaged heart tissue. Bacteria are the cause of most cases, but fungi or other microorganisms also may be responsible.

Sometimes the culprit is one of many common bacteria that live in the mouth, upper respiratory tract, or other parts of the body. In other cases, the offending organism may gain entry to the bloodstream through:

- Common activities. Everyday activities such as brushing teeth or chewing food can allow bacteria to enter the bloodstream, especially if the teeth and gums are in poor condition.
- An infection or other medical condition. Bacteria may spread from an infected area, such as a skin sore. Gum disease, a sexually transmitted disease, or an intestinal disorder, such as inflammatory bowel disease, also may give bacteria the opportunity to enter the bloodstream.
- Catheters or needles. Bacteria can enter the body through a catheter, a thin tube that doctors sometimes use to inject or remove fluid from the body. Contaminated needles and syringes are a concern for people who use intravenous (IV) drugs.
- Certain dental or respiratory tract procedures. Some dental procedures may allow bacteria to enter the bloodstream.

Typically, the immune system destroys bacteria that make it into the bloodstream. Even if bacteria reach the heart, they may pass through without causing an infection.

Most people who develop endocarditis have a diseased or damaged heart valve, an ideal spot for bacteria to settle. This damaged tissue in the endocardium provides bacteria with the roughened surface they need to attach and multiply.

Even most types of heart disease don't increase the risk

of endocarditis. The organisms that cause infection tend to adhere to and multiply only in malformed, damaged, or surgically implanted heart valves.

Those at highest risk of endocarditis are those who have:

- Artificial heart valves. Germs are more likely to attach to an artificial (prosthetic) heart valve than a normal heart valve. The risk of infection is highest in the first year after implantation.
- Congenital heart defects. If the patient was born with certain types of heart defects, such as mitral valve prolapse, the heart may be more susceptible to infection.
- A prior history of endocarditis. An episode of endocarditis damages heart tissue and valves, increasing the risk of a future heart infection.
- Damaged heart valves. Certain medical conditions, such as rheumatic fever or infection, can damage or scar one or more of the heart valves, making them more prone to endocarditis.

Some people without heart problems are at risk of endocarditis as well. Intravenous drug users have a greater risk of infection because sharing or reusing needles can expose the bloodstream to infectious agents. People who are hospitalized with IV tubes also may be exposed to infection.

The doctor may suspect endocarditis based on medical history and physical signs and symptoms, such as fever. Using a stethoscope to listen to the heart, the doctor may hear a new heart murmur or a change in a previous heart murmur, possible signs of endocarditis. The infection can mimic other illnesses in its early stages. Various tests may be necessary to help make the diagnosis.

Endocarditis can cause clumps of bacteria and cellular debris (vegetations) to form in the heart at the site of the infection. These clumps can break loose and travel to the brain, lungs, abdominal organs, or kidneys. This may cause various problems, including stroke or damage to other organs.

Left untreated, endocarditis can damage the heart valves and permanently destroy the heart's inner lining. This can cause the heart to work harder to pump blood, eventually causing heart failure, a chronic condition in which the heart is unable to pump enough blood to meet the body's needs. If the infection progresses untreated, it's usually fatal.

To treat endocarditis, the patient will need high doses of intravenous antibiotics in the hospital. Blood tests will help identify the type of microorganism that's infecting the heart. The patient will need to take antibiotics orally for at least six weeks after discharge from hospital to clear up the infection.

If the infection damages the heart valves, the patient may have symptoms and complications for years after treatment. Sometimes surgery is needed to treat persistent infections or replace a damaged valve.

Meningitis: Bacterial and Viral

Meningitis is an inflammation of the meninges, the lining of the spinal cord and brain beneath the skull. Bacteria or a virus can cause it. Meningitis is more common in children than adults.

Bacterial meningitis is bacteria (pneumoccal and meningococcal are the most common) that cause meningitis. It normally lives in the back of our noses and throats. Most people who have these germs do not even know it, as they do not become ill. However, some people, for reasons that doctors do not understand, do get sick from these germs. Other people get meningitis from germs that cause ear infections or other minor illnesses when they get into the blood and/or area around the brain and spinal cord.

Viral meningitis is more common than bacterial. It is caused by many different viruses; enteroviruses are the most common and usually occur in the summer and early fall.

A common way of spreading both the bacterial and viral germs is through human saliva. This includes sharing food, drinking from the same glass, and kissing. The germs are also spread through coughing, sneezing, or poor hygiene. Regular hand washing with soap, water, and friction for ten to fifteen seconds is a great way of preventing these germs from being spread.

Symptoms of meningitis are much like having the flu. They include fussiness or irritability, weakness, tiredness, not eating or drinking as much, vomiting, fever, and headache. More serious signs may be a bulging soft spot (in infants), a stiff neck, bright lights hurting the eyes, a small pinpoint rash (purple or blood-red in color), confusion, and seizures (convulsions).

Bacterial meningitis is more severe than viral meningitis and is potentially life threatening. Antibiotics will be needed to clear up the meningitis. Viral meningitis does not need antibiotics to cure it and is rarely life threatening. It will run its course like the flu.

It may be difficult to tell the difference between bacterial and viral meningitis at first. A blood test and lumbar puncture (spinal tap) must be done to find out what type of meningitis a child has. A patient with either type may be given antibiotics at first. Intravenous antibiotics may be used to treat the child because the medications given this way work best. These antibiotics will be started as soon as possible after the tests are obtained.

While someone has meningitis, the room should be kept quiet and as dark as possible. Sometimes bacterial meningitis can damage hearing, so after the patient feels better, a hearing test may be done.

Meningitis is hard to prevent, but great measures are being taken to stop this disease. HIB (haemophilus influenza type b) meningitis was the most common bacterial form in infants. This meningitis is now very rare because of the HIB vaccine that is part of routine immunizations.

As previously stated, frequent hand washing with soap and water vigorously for ten to fifteen seconds is the best way to stop the spread of meningitis. Not sharing body fluids through cups, straws, eating utensils, or kissing is also necessary to keep in mind for prevention of meningitis.

Methicillin-Resistant Staphylococcus Aureus (MRSA)

MRSA stands for methicillin-resistant Staphylococcus aureus. It is a type of bacterium commonly found on the skin and/or in the noses of healthy people. Although it is usually harmless at these sites, it may occasionally get into the body through breaks in the skin, such as abrasions, cuts, wounds, surgical incisions, or indwelling catheters, and cause infections. These infections may be mild pimples or boils or a serious infection of the bloodstream, bones, or joints.

The treatment of infections due to Staphylococcus aureus was revolutionized in the 1940s by the introduction of the antibiotic penicillin. Unfortunately, most strains of Staphylococcus aureus are now resistant to penicillin.

MRSA infections most often occur in patients in hospitals and are becoming more commonly seen among the general public. As with ordinary strains of Staphylococcus aureus, some patients harbor MRSA on their skin or nose without harm (such patients are said to be colonized), and other patients may develop infections.

Some patients are at increased risk of developing infection. They include those with breaks in their skin due to wounds including those caused by surgery, indwelling catheters or burns, and those with certain types of deficiencies in their immune system, such as low numbers of white cells in their blood.

In addition to causing endogenous infections, MRSA can spread between patients, usually by direct or indirect physical contact. For example, hospital staff attending to a colonized or infected patient may become contaminated or colonized with MRSA themselves (perhaps only briefly). They may then spread the bacteria to other patients with whom they subsequently have contact. These patients may in turn become colonized and/or infected. The spread of MRSA (or for that matter other bacteria) between patients is called cross-infection.

To diagnose MRSA infections, specimens are taken from the patient, such as a swab of an infected wound or a sample of blood or urine. These are sent to a microbiology laboratory, where bacteria present in the specimen are cultured and identified. This process may take several days. Colonization with MRSA is detected similarly, using swabs of a person's skin or from the inside of the nose.

Patients colonized with MRSA and patients infected with MRSA are treated differently. Patients or other individuals simply colonized with MRSA may have a special antibiotic called mupirocin applied onto their skin (Bactroban) or the inside of their nose (Bactroban nasal). This helps to eliminate the MRSA and reduces the risk of the bacteria spreading either to other sites on the patient's body, where they might cause infection, or to other patients. Some strains of MRSA are, however, resistant to mupirocin. Individuals colonized with MRSA may also wash their skin and hair with suitable disinfectants such as chlorhexidine.

Patients with infections due to Staphylococcus aureus often need antibiotics. Infections due to normal strains of Staphylococcus aureus are often treated with flucloxacillin (Floxapen), but this is ineffective against MRSA. To make matters worse, MRSA are often also resistant to other types of antibiotics such as erythromycin (Erythroped) and ciprofloxacin (Ciproxin).

Staph is the usual suspect in many skin infections. Staph

infections, including those caused by MRSA, usually begin as red bumps resembling boils or pimples. (People sometimes mistake them for spider bites.) The bumps often become swollen, painful, and filled with pus.

Most staph skin infections are often minor and can be remedied by regularly washing and bandaging the area and/or using oral antibiotics or antibiotic ointments. Sometimes the abscesses from staph need to be drained by a doctor.

But MRSA can't be treated with antibiotics that are routinely given, such as methicillin, penicillin, and amoxicillin. Doctors now have turned to other medications to try to treat MRSA. And, if the infection spreads to other parts of the body, MRSA may lead to serious complications, like pneumonia and blood and joint infections.

MRSA is affecting more people outside of hospitals. MRSA used to be seen only in those with weakened immune systems, chronically ill people who'd been hospitalized for a long time or had surgery, those receiving long courses of antibiotic therapy, or people living in long-term-care facilities like nursing homes or prisons.

But now an alarming number of otherwise healthy people who are not considered at risk for MRSA are getting the infection. Called community-associated MRSA (or CA-MRSA), this type of staph infection has been found most recently in a few high school and professional sports teams. The bug can be passed to athletes via gyms and locker rooms and through shared equipment or skin-to-skin contact (e.g., wrestling and football). Kids in childcare settings may also be at risk.

Staph infections can spread through the air and to

other people or other parts of your body via contaminated surfaces or on dirty hands or fingernails. To help keep the super-bug at bay in your household:

- Make sure every member of your family washes his or her hands well and often
- Use alcohol-based instant hand sanitizers
- Keep any broken skin clean and covered with a bandage
- Don't share razors or towels
- Make sure shared sports equipment is cleaned with antiseptic solution before each use

Call the doctor if:

- The child has an area of skin that is red, painful, swollen, and/or filled with pus
- The child has inflamed skin and is also feverish or feels sick
- Skin infections seem to be passing from one family member to another, or if two or more family members have skin infections at the same time

Serious cases of MRSA are still relatively rare, but an ounce of prevention can go a long way toward avoiding the infection and keeping your family healthy.

Sepsis

Sepsis is an infection in the bloodstream. Babies have immature immune systems, which means they are unable to fight infections as well as older children and adults. Infections in newborns are usually caused by bacteria or viruses.

Decreased heart rate (bradycardia), decreased or absent breathing (apnea), pale or gray color, decreased level of activity, increased or decreased temperature, and feeding intolerance are some of the symptoms that would be seen in an infant that is septic. Medically fragile infants are susceptible to sepsis, and it is very important that you are familiar with the infant in your care.

Tests will be done to find out what is causing the infection. These tests may include blood or urine cultures, sputum cultures, spinal fluid cultures, and X-rays. Antibiotics will be started. Other treatments are given based on the baby's symptoms. For example, the baby may need extra oxygen or help breathing.

Most babies who have an infection will stay on antibiotics for seven to ten days. Usually they feel better within a few days of starting the antibiotics, but it is very important that they take the full treatment of antibiotics to prevent the infection from coming back. The most important thing you can do is to get to know the baby that you are caring for so that you can recognize when he or she acts differently.

Vancomycin-Resistant Enterococci (VRE)

Enteroccocci are bacteria that are normally present in the human intestines and in the female genital tract and are often found in the environment. These bacteria can sometimes cause infections. Vancomycin is an antibiotic that is often used to treat infections caused by enterococci. In some instances, enterococci have become resistant to this drug and thus are called vancomycin resistant enterococci (VRE). Most VRE infections occur in hospitals.

VRE can live in the human intestines and female genital tract without causing disease. However, sometimes it can be the cause of urinary tract infections, bloodstream infections, and wound infections.

The following persons are at an increased risk of becoming infected with VRE:

- Persons who have been previously treated with vancomycin and combinations of other antibiotics such as penicillin and gentamicin
- Persons who are hospitalized, particularly when they receive antibiotic treatment for long periods of time
- Persons with weakened immune systems, such as patients in intensive care units or in cancer or transplant wards
- Persons who have undergone surgical procedures such as abdominal or chest surgery
- Persons with medical devices that stay in for some time, such as urinary catheters or central intravenous catheters

Most VRE infections can be treated with antibiotics other than vancomycin. The treatment of VRE is determined by laboratory testing to determine which antibiotics are effective. For persons who get VRE infections and have urinary catheters, removal of the catheter when it is no longer needed could help get rid of the infection. People who are colonized (bacteria are present, but have no symptoms of an infection) with VRE do not usually need treatment.

VRE is usually passed to others by direct contact with stool, urine, or blood containing VRE. It can also be spread indirectly via the hands of health-care providers or on contaminated environmental surfaces. VRE usually is not spread through casual contact such as touching or hugging. VRE is not spread through the air by coughing or sneezing.

If you or someone in your household has VRE, the following are some measures to prevent spread of VRE:

- Always wash your hands thoroughly after using the bathroom and before preparing food. Clean your hands after close contact with persons who have VRE. Wash with soap and water (particularly when visibly soiled) or clean with alcohol-based hand cleaner.
- Frequently clean areas of your home, such as your bathroom, that may become contaminated with VRE. Use a household disinfectant or a mixture of one-fourth cup of bleach and one quart of water to clean those areas and surfaces that are touched frequently.
- Wear gloves if you may come in contact with body fluids that may contain VRE, such as stool. Always wash your hands after removing gloves.

- Be sure to tell any health-care providers that you or the child that you are caring for has VRE so that they are aware of the infection.

VRE is not dangerous in healthy people with strong immune systems, where the balance of healthy flora in their digestive tract helps keep VRE from getting out of control.

VRE is dangerous because it cannot be controlled with antibiotics, and it causes life-threatening infections in people with compromised immune systems: the very young, the very old, and the very ill. It is especially dangerous because it can easily transmit the resistance genes to other, more dangerous bacteria, such as staph and strep. These could cause serious infections even in otherwise healthy people. You can be exposed to VRE by coming in contact with a contaminated object or person or by eating contaminated food.

VRE has been cultured from hospital equipment, doorknobs, and bedrails. It has also been cultured on the hands of hospital personnel. Anyone who frequents hospitals should be considered at risk for carrying VRE. Fastidious hygiene is the best way to avoid ingesting VRE and becoming a carrier. VRE is a robust bacterium and has been found on hospital personnel's hands after five seconds of hand washing. It is recommended that you wash your hands for twenty seconds with an antibacterial soap every time before you eat.

Neurological Disorders

Cerebral Palsy

Cerebral palsy (CP) is a nonprogressive, neuromuscular disorder of varying degrees resulting from damage or developmental defects in the part of the brain that controls motor function.

Children with CP can't control movements in certain parts of their bodies and may be partially paralyzed. They may have completely normal intelligence and may feel as if they're trapped in a body they can't control.

Conditions that result in cerebral anoxia, hemorrhage, or other damage are probably responsible for CP.

Prenatal conditions that may increase the risk of CP include maternal infection (especially rubella), maternal drug ingestion, radiation, anoxia, toxemia, maternal diabetes, abnormal placental attachment, malnutrition, and isoimmunization.

Perinatal and birth difficulties that increase the risk of CP include forceps delivery, breech presentation, placenta previa, abruptio placentae, metabolic or electrolyte disturbances, abnormal maternal vital signs from general or spinal anesthetic, prolapsed cord with delay in delivery of the head, premature birth, prolonged or unusually rapid labor, and multiple birth (especially infants born last in a multiple birth).

Infection or trauma during infancy that increases the risk of CP includes poisoning, severe kernicterus resulting from erythroblastosis fetalis, brain infection, head trauma, prolonged anoxia, brain tumor, cerebral circulatory anomalies causing blood vessel rupture, and systemic disease resulting in cerebral thrombosis or embolus.

There are three distinct types of CP:

- Spastic
- Athetoid
- Ataxic

Spastic CP is the most common type, affecting about 70 percent of CP patients. The affected area of the brain is the cortex. Typically, the child with spastic CP walks on his toes with a scissor gait, crossing one foot in front of the other.

Spastic CP is characterized by:

- Increased deep tendon reflexes
- Hypertonia
- Flexion
- Tendency to have contractures
- Rapid involuntary muscle contraction and relaxation
- Underdevelopment of affected limbs.

In athetoid CP, which affects about 20 percent of CP patients, involuntary, uncoordinated motion occurs with varying degrees of muscle tension. The area of injury is the basal ganglia. The child exhibits slow, writhing, uncontrolled movements involving all extremities whenever voluntary movement is attempted. Facial grimacing, poor swallowing, and drooling make speech difficult.

Ataxic CP accounts for about 10 percent of CP patients. The affected area of the brain is the cerebellum. Its characteristics include poor balance and muscle coordination caused by disturbances in movement and balance. An unsteady, wide-based gait appears as the child begins to learn to walk; overall, the child appears clumsy.

Some children with CP display a combination of these clinical features:

- In most, delayed gross motor development makes eating, especially swallowing, difficult.
- Abnormal motor performance and coordination can manifest early in life as poor sucking and feeding difficulty.
- Spasticity of hip muscles and lower extremities makes diapering difficult.
- Posture abnormalities occur at rest or when changing position.
- Mental retardation occurs in varying degrees in 18 percent to 50 percent of patients (most children with CP have an IQ that is normal or higher, but they can't demonstrate it on standardized tests).
- Seizures occur in 25 percent of CP patients.
- Many children have sensory deficits related to vision (strabismus), hearing, and speech.

What the different tests can tell you:

- Developmental screening reveals delay in achieving milestones.
- EEG may identify the source of seizure activity.
- Neuroimaging studies (CT scan, MRI) determine the site of brain impairment.
- Cytogenic studies (genetic evaluation of the child and other family members) and metabolic studies are performed to rule out other potential causes.

Children with CP may also have associated disorders such as impaired intellectual development, seizures, failure to grow and thrive, and problems with vision and sense of touch.

CP can't be cured, but proper treatment can help affected children reach their full potential within the limitations set by this disorder. Treatment includes the following:

- A baclofen (Lioresal) pump may be inserted to treat spasticity by delivering the skeletal muscle relaxant directly to the intrathecal space around the spinal cord. (The pump lasts for three to five years, after which a new pump must be implanted.)
- Oral muscle relaxants may be used or neurosurgery may be required to decrease spasticity.
- Braces or splints and special appliances, such as adapted eating utensils and a low toilet seat with arms, can help the child perform activities independently.

- Range of Motion (ROM) exercises minimize contractures.
- An artificial urinary sphincter may be recommended for the incontinent child who is able to use hand controls.
- Orthopedic surgery may be suggested to correct contractures.
- Phenytoin (Dilantin), phenobarbital (Bellatal), or another anticonvulsant may be used to control seizures.

Care of the child with CP involves attention to diet and physical activity.

- A high-calorie diet may be instituted with a doctor's input for the child with increased motor function to help him keep up with increased metabolic demands.
- Assist with locomotion, communication, and educational opportunities to enable the child to attain an optimal developmental level.
- Perform ROM exercises to minimize contractures.
- Plan activities that involve gross and fine motor skills, such as holding toys or eating utensils and positioning items to encourage reaching and rolling over.
- Provide a safe environment; have the child use protective headgear or bed pads to prevent injury.

Hydrocephalus

Hydrocephalus means an enlargement of the ventricles in the brain. This is caused by an obstruction of the flow of the cerebrospinal fluid.

Hydrocephalus may exist before birth, or something can happen after birth, such as an infection in the brain or bleeding in the brain. The fluid will build up and cause the ventricles to enlarge. If the ventricles continue to enlarge, the brain tissue will be compressed. Sometimes hydrocephalus will stop, and surgery is not needed. If it does not stop on its own, a thin tube called a shunt is inserted through the brain into the ventricle; the other part of the tube is passed beneath the skin into the abdominal cavity. This is called a ventriculoperitoneal shunt (VP shunt). This shunt will drain the cerebrospinal fluid into the abdomen where it is reabsorbed when it starts to build up. The baby will probably need the shunt all his life. He may need to have the shunt replaced because of growth and possible problems.

In infants, the unmistakable sign of hydrocephalus is the enlargement of the head clearly disproportionate to the infant's growth. Other characteristic changes include distended scalp veins; thin, fragile, and shiny-looking scalp skin; and underdeveloped neck muscles. In severe cases, the eyes are displaced downward, and the sclera is prominent (sunset eyes, setting-sun sign). A high-pitched, shrill cry, abnormal muscle tone of the legs, irritability, anorexia, and projectile vomiting often occur.

There are several tests that can be done to diagnose hydrocephalus, and these are as follows:

- Head ultrasound (HUS): Takes a picture of the baby's brain using sound waves. A sensor is placed over the soft spot on the head. Sound waves measure the brain tissue, and a picture is made. This does not hurt the baby.
- CAT Scan (computerized axial tomography): Uses a beam of X-ray to take pictures of the brain. The baby will go inside a large machine, and he must be still for the test. Oftentimes, medication is given to make baby sleepy for the test. The test does not hurt the baby.
- MRI (magnetic resonance imaging): This test is similar to the CAT scan; however, it uses magnetic rays as opposed to X-rays. The baby must be very still for this test and usually needs medication to help him sleep. This test does not hurt the baby.

The major complications of VP shunts are infection and malfunction. All shunts are subject to mechanical difficulties such as kinking, plugging, or separation or migration of the tubing. Malfunction is most often caused by mechanical obstruction either within the ventricles from particulate matter (tissue or exudate) or at the distal end from thrombosis or displacement because of growth.

The most serious complication, shunt infection, can occur at any time, but the period of greatest risk is one to two months following placement. An infection is treated with massive doses of antibiotics administered by the intravenous route or directly into the ventricles via the shunt reservoir. A persistent infection requires removal of the shunt until the infection is controlled.

The following assessment findings indicate shunt malfunction or infection:

- Swelling along shunt tract
- High-pitched cry
- Bulging fontanels
- Prominent scalp veins
- Irritability when awake
- Increased frontal occipital circumference
- Projectile vomiting
- Change in appetite
- Lethargy
- Lower extremity spasticity
- Elevated temperature

The infant with a shunt obstruction or infection often presents as an emergency with clinical manifestations of increased intracranial pressure, frequently accompanied by worsening neurologic status.

The outcome of hydrocephalus depends on the cause, the part of the brain involved, and the severity of the problem. While many hydrocephalic children have neurological problems, some are normal. It is important for the baby to be seen by a doctor who specializes in infant development.

Intraventricular Hemorrhage

Intraventricular hemorrhage (IVH) means bleeding into the normal fluid spaces (ventricles) within the brain. IVH is also used to refer to bleeding in areas near the ventricles even if the blood is not within them.

The extent of IVH is graded.

- Grade I: bleeding confined to the tiny area where it first begins
- Grade II: blood is also within the ventricles
- Grade III: more extensive bleeding, usually with the ventricles increasing in size
- Grade IV: a collection of blood within the substance of the brain, also called intraparenchymal echodensities because of its appearance on the ultrasound picture. This can be seen with Grade I, II, or III IVH.

With the premature infant, the brain is still developing. The area where IVH usually begins has a very fragile group of tiny blood vessels. These burst easily, causing the bleeding. The more premature and the sicker the baby is, the greater the risk that he or she will develop IVH. The infants at highest risk are those weighing less than one thousand grams (2 1/4 pounds).

Most of the time there are no outward signs that the bleeding has occurred; occasionally babies have seizures or sudden anemia. Babies at significant risk for IVH usually have an ultrasound of the head in the first three to ten days of life. This painless test, performed in the isolette or bed, uses sound waves to give a picture of the baby's brain. If IVH is present, the baby may have this test repeated at regular intervals to see if the hemorrhage or the size of the ventricles is increasing.

There is no specific treatment for IVH.

Complications are most common with grades III and IV IVH. The most frequent complication of IVH is hydrocephalus, or too much fluid collecting in the ventricles. This extra fluid may cause the baby's head to grow more rapidly than normal or pressure on the baby's brain.

Grades I and II IVH are most common. They usually do not cause brain injury. The blood is slowly absorbed by the body. Babies with Grade III IVH are at increased risk of brain damage, but most are normal or near normal. Babies who have needed treatment for hydrocephalus and those with grade IV IVH are at highest risk for permanent brain injury. Long-term problems can only be determined over time by monitoring his or her development. For this reason, it is important for premature infants, especially those with Grade III through IV IVH, to have their development followed carefully after discharge.

Serious abnormalities that may appear are:

- Motor (movement) problems: tight or stiff muscles; slow to crawl, stand, or walk; abnormal crawling; toe walking; moving one side more than the other; frequent arching of the back (not just when angry or at play).
- Slow mental development: does not listen to

your voice by age three to four months, does not make different sounds by eight to nine months, doesn't seem to understand or say any words by twelve to thirteen months.

- Seizures.

Less serious problems appear more slowly, are more difficult to detect, and may not be obvious until preschool or grade school. These can include:

- Poor coordination or balance
- Specific learning disabilities (math or reading)
- Very short attention span
- Behavioral problems
- Difficulty with activities that require coordination of the eyes and hands, for example, catching a ball or copying a simple drawing

Neonatal Encephalopathy

Neonatal encephalopathy is a heterogeneous syndrome characterized by symptoms of central nervous system dysfunction in newborns born at or near term. An infant with neonatal encephalopathy may exhibit an abnormal level of consciousness, seizures, tone and reflex abnormalities, apnea, and feeding difficulties. Researchers have yet to adopt a consensus of definition of neonatal encephalopathy.

Neonatal encephalopathy can result from a wide variety of conditions and often remains unexplained. Birth asphyxia and hypoxic-ischemic encephalopathy are responsible for some, but not all, cases of neonatal encephalopathy. Given that the underlying nature of brain injury causing neurologic impairment in a newborn is often poorly understood, neonatal encephalopathy has emerged as the preferred terminology to describe central nervous system dysfunction in the newborn period, as it does not imply a specific underlying pathophysiology.

The neonate who is encephalopathic may have an abnormal state of consciousness (e.g., hyperalert, irritable, lethargic, obtunded), respiratory or feeding difficulties, poor tone, or seizure activity. In the delivery room, the infant will often exhibit low Apgar scores and a weak or absent cry.

Seizures

Seizures are a short-circuiting of the brain's electrical impulses. Seizures occur most often when brain tissue is irritated or injured. Conditions that can cause seizures are metabolic imbalances, bleeding in the brain, meningitis, brain edema, and some drug withdrawals. Seizures in an infant are sometimes hard to detect from normal premature behaviors; it may be trembling of the mouth, fluttering of the eyelids, rolling of the eyes, flailing of the arms and legs (especially if it can't be stopped), and also apnea and bradycardia. Usually an EEG (electroencephalogram), a brain-wave tracing, is used to make the diagnosis. It is very important that seizures are treated. The brain cells require huge amounts of sugar and oxygen during a seizure; when these needs are not met, brain cells can die. Medications are given to control seizures. Depending on the cause of the seizures, medication may be necessary for a few weeks, months, or indefinitely. Seizures frequently involve apnea. There are several different types of seizures.

Although the primary management of seizures is the responsibility of the physician, the teachers, facility staff, and parents play an important role in monitoring the frequency and duration of the seizures. Giving the anticonvulsant medication as directed by the physician and monitoring the child for the appearance of possible side effects of any medications is everyone's responsibility. Staff, teachers, and parents should recognize the various types of seizures, as well as information regarding the various, frequently prescribed anticonvulsant medications.

Types of seizures:

- Grand mal seizures consist of a loss of consciousness accompanied by uncontrolled muscle contractions over the whole body. Movements typically consist of jerking of the arms and legs and rolling of the eyes to one side. This is frequently accompanied by loss of bowel and/or bladder control and difficulty breathing. The seizure typically lasts several minutes and is followed by a period of sleepiness and confusion lasting an hour or more.
- Petit mal seizures consist of a very brief lapse of consciousness, usually accompanied by eye blinking or other facial movements. Posture is maintained, and the individual continues on as if nothing happened. There is a typical brain

wave pattern on the EEG. These seizures can be differentiated from daydreaming by attempting to capture the attention of the individual by saying a high-interest word such as McDonald's or Mutant Ninja Turtles. If the individual stops staring but does not remember what was said, this may have been a petit mal seizure and should be reported to the physician. If this occurs several times in a day, the frequency and duration should be noted and conveyed to the medical providers.

- Atypical absence (Lenox Gastaut syndrome) seizures consist of atypical staring spells, sometimes accompanied by violent contractions of one or more muscle groups. This may result in a fall. This type of seizure is very difficult to control and is generally accompanied by mental retardation.
- Simple partial (focal) seizures consist of jerking of one part of the body, but consciousness is unimpaired. This type of seizure may spread and become a grand mal. It is frequently an indicator of severe neurological disease and has a poorer prognosis than many others.
- Partial complex (psychomotor) seizures consist of an alteration of consciousness accompanied by a fixed pattern of movement that mimic some natural movements, such as sitting, running, or atypical speech. The automatisms that occur during the period of lost consciousness associated with complex particle seizures can have the appearance of aggressive action. Because the patient is unconscious when these occur, however, these behaviors are not under the patient's

> control and are not intended to be harmful. The patient will not remember the behaviors after becoming fully conscious. Automatisms occur at sometime or other in more than three out of four children with complex partial seizures, particularly those with a temporal lobe focus.

The automatisms that occur during seizures consist of a wide range of poorly coordinated, semipurposeful activities and vary widely among patients but tend to be stereotyped from one seizure to another in each child. It is easy to see how a patient who is thrashing, yelling, and resisting restraint would be characterized by many observers as demonstrating aggressive behavior. In addition, automatisms can occur during the postictal phase of seizures while the patient is still significantly confused.

The postictal phase is the period following a seizure when alertness and mental activity is diminished. If the patient is physically restrained during this time, he or she may react with aggressive behavior against the restraining person. If left alone, except for maneuvers to protect the patient's safety, there will most likely be no directed violence. The importance of adequate baseline data cannot be overemphasized. Good observational data on the frequency, intensity, and duration of outbursts, with good descriptive data, is critical in assessing whenever seizure activity is suspected. These assessments will provide information about the effectiveness of medical interventions and/or medications.

Shaken Baby Syndrome

Shaken baby syndrome (SBS) is a form of inflicted head trauma. Head injury is a form of child abuse that can be caused by direct blows to the head, dropping or throwing the child, or shaking the child. Head trauma is the leading cause of death in child abuse cases in the United States.

Unlike other forms of inflicted head trauma, SBS results from injuries caused by someone vigorously shaking an infant. Because of the anatomy of infants, they're at particular risk for injury from this kind of action. Therefore, the vast majority of incidents occur in infants who are younger than one year old. The average age of victims is between three and eight months, although SBS is occasionally seen in children up to four years old.

The perpetrators in SBS cases are almost always parents or caregivers who shake the baby out of frustration or stress when the little one is crying inconsolably. Sadly, the shaking has the desired effect. Although at first the baby cries more out of fear, it eventually stops crying, as the brain is damaged.

When someone forcefully shakes a baby, the child's head rotates about uncontrollably because infants' neck muscles aren't well developed and provide little support for their heads. The violent movement pitches the infant's brain back and forth within the skull, rupturing blood vessels and nerves throughout the brain and tearing the brain tissue. The brain strikes the inside of the skull, causing bruising and bleeding to the brain.

The damage is even greater when the shaking ends with an impact (hitting a wall or a crib mattress, for example), because the forces of acceleration and deceleration associated with an impact are so strong. After the shaking, swelling in the brain can cause enormous pressure within the skull, compressing blood vessels and increasing overall injury to its delicate structure.

Normal interaction with a child, like bouncing a baby on a knee, will not cause SBS, although it's important never to shake a baby under any circumstances because gentle shaking can rapidly escalate. SBS often causes irreversible damage. In the worst cases, the death rate is almost half of all babies involved.

Children who survive may have:

- Partial or total blindness
- Hearing loss
- Seizures
- Developmental delays
- Impaired intellect
- Speech and learning difficulties
- Problems with memory and attention
- Severe mental retardation
- Paralysis (some particularly traumatic episodes leave children in a coma)

Even in milder cases in which babies look normal immediately after the shaking, they may eventually develop one or more of these problems.

Sometimes the first sign of a problem isn't noticed until

the child enters the school system and exhibits behavioral problems or learning difficulties. But by that time, it's more difficult to link these problems to a shaking incident from several years before.

In any SBS case, the duration and force of the shaking, the number of episodes, and whether impact is involved all affect the severity of the infant's injuries. In the most violent cases, children may arrive at the emergency room unconscious, suffering seizures, or in shock. But in many cases, infants may never be brought to medical attention if they don't exhibit such severe symptoms.

In less severe cases, a baby who has been shaken may experience:

- Lethargy
- Irritability
- Vomiting
- Poor sucking or swallowing
- Decreased appetite
- Lack of smiling or vocalizing
- Rigidity
- Seizures
- Difficulty breathing
- Altered consciousness
- Unequal pupil size
- An inability to lift the head
- An inability to focus the eyes or track movement

Many cases of SBS are brought in for medical care as silent injuries. In other words, parents or caregivers don't often provide a history that the child has had abusive head trauma or a shaking injury, so doctors don't know to look for subtle physical signs. This silent epidemic can result in children having injuries that aren't identified in the medical system.

And again, in many cases, babies who don't have severe symptoms may never be brought to a doctor.

Unfortunately, unless a doctor has reason to suspect SBS, mild cases (in which the infant seems lethargic, fussy, or perhaps isn't feeding well) are often misdiagnosed as a viral illness or colic. Without a diagnosis of shaken baby syndrome and any resulting intervention with the parents or caregivers, these children may be shaken again, worsening any brain injury or damage.

If shaken baby syndrome is suspected, doctors may look for:

- Hemorrhages in the retinas of the eyes (which are extremely rare in any accidental injuries, such as falls)
- Skull fractures
- Swelling of the brain
- Subdural hematomas (blood collections pressing on the surface of the brain)
- Rib and long bone (bones in the arms and legs) fractures
- Bruises around the head, neck, or chest

What makes SBS so devastating is that it usually involves a total brain injury. Because the infant's immature brain has little stored information and few developed capacities to make up for the deficit, the brain's adaptive abilities are substantially impaired. For example, a child whose vision is severely impaired won't be able to learn through observation, which decreases the child's overall ability to learn.

The development of language, vision, balance, and motor coordination, all of which occur to varying degrees after birth, are particularly likely to be affected in any child who has SBS.

Such impairment can require rigorous physical and occupational therapy to help the child acquire skills that would have developed on his or her own had the brain injury not occurred. Therapists do this by providing a sensory-rich environment, which forces the child to be attentive.

Shaken baby syndrome is one-hundred-percent preventable.

A key aspect of prevention of the syndrome is increasing awareness of the potential dangers of shaking. Some hospital-based programs have helped new parents identify and prevent shaking injuries and understand how to respond when infants cry. Finding ways to alleviate the parent or caregiver's stress at the critical moments when a baby is crying can significantly reduce the risk to the child. If a baby in your care won't stop crying, you can try the following:

- Make sure the baby's basic needs are met (for example, he or she isn't hungry and doesn't need to be changed)

- Check for signs of illness, like fever or swollen gums
- Swaddling (wrapping the baby up snugly in a blanket to help him or her feel more secure)
- Rock or walk with the baby
- Sing or talk to the baby
- Offer the baby a pacifier or a noisy toy
- Take the baby for a ride in a stroller or strapped into a child safety seat in the car
- Hold the baby close against your body and breathe calmly and slowly
- Call a friend or relative for support or to take care of the baby while you take a break
- If nothing else works, put the baby on his or her back in the crib, close the door, and check on the baby in ten minutes.
- Call your child's doctor if nothing seems to be helping your infant in case there is a medical reason for the fussiness

To prevent potential SBS, parents and caregivers of infants need help with responding to their own stress. It's important to talk to anyone caring for your baby about the dangers of shaking and how it can be prevented.

Respiratory Disorders

Asthma

Asthma is a chronic, inflammatory lung disease characterized by recurrent breathing problems. Infants with asthma have acute episodes when the air passages in their lungs get narrower, and breathing becomes more difficult. These problems are caused by an oversensitivity of the lungs and airways, which overreact to certain triggers and become inflamed and clogged. Asthma attacks can strike without warning and last from minutes to days. There is no cure for asthma, but asthma can be controlled with proper treatment. Symptoms may be as subtle as a hacking cough or chest tightness or as severe as a life-threatening inability to breathe.

Typically, symptoms include:

- Wheezing, the whistling sound caused by air moving through the narrowed airway
- Breathlessness, the result of too many swollen, plugged-up airways
- Coughing, the lungs' attempt to dislodge the mucus

Most asthma medications fall into one of two categories. Bronchodilators offer quick relief by relaxing the muscles that keep air from flowing into the lungs. Their action opens blocked airways. Anti-inflammatories help prevent attacks by making the airways less reactive to triggers so they do not swell. These latter medications need to be taken regularly even if no symptoms are present.

Asthma is a lung disease that can be treated. Asthma can be very different from one person to another and from one episode (attack) to another. For some, asthma causes only mild symptoms occasionally. For others, every day can be a struggle to breathe. Some asthma attacks last only a few minutes; others go on for days. Some asthma attacks are just a bother. Others quickly become life threatening.

The most common symptoms of asthma are:

- Recurrent wheezing (a whistling or hissing sound as you breathe out)
- Recurrent shortness of breath
- Recurrent feeling of tightness in the chest
- A cough that lasts for more than a week

Not all people with asthma wheeze. For some, coughing, especially during the night or after exercise, may be the main symptom.

Three changes occur inside the airways in the lungs of people with asthma. The first change is inflammation (or swelling) that leads to the next two changes: constriction and sensitivity.

- Inflammation: The tissues inside the airways can easily become inflamed (redness, irritation, or swelling). The inflamed tissues make thick mucus. In addition, if inflammation happens often and is severe, it causes permanent thickening of the tissues in the airways.

- Constriction: The muscles around the airways are likely to constrict (tighten), causing the airways to become narrow. This is also called bronchospasm or bronchoconstriction.
- Sensitivity: The airways are overly sensitive to animal dander, pollen, tobacco smoke, air pollution, the common cold, or even cold air.

During an asthma episode (attack), these three airway changes (inflammation, constriction, and sensitivity) get worse at the same time, and this causes problems.

- Airways swell on the inside and constrict from the outside. This blocks the flow of air.
- Thick mucus plugs the smaller airways.
- Breathing becomes a struggle.
- Whistling or wheezing sounds may start.
- The chest feels tight.
- The individual may cough as he or she tries to clear the lungs.

Prevention and education are the best medicine. You need to know how asthma affects the child's airways in order to know how you can control it. The best asthma attack is the one that does not happen!

Asthma treatment has two goals:

- Keeping symptoms from starting in the first place. The best way to do this is to always follow the child's treatment plan that the physician has developed. You need to follow the plan, if necessary, even when the child does not have any asthma symptoms.
- Spotting symptoms that are getting worse before they get bad. This allows you to treat the symptoms early, when they are easiest to control.

Tools for Self-Management of Asthma

- Know the basic facts of asthma
- Know the roles of medications
- Learn the skills involved with the use of inhaled medications and use of peak flow meters
- Control the things that trigger an asthma attack
- Know when and how to administer medicines for asthma attacks, and be sure the child knows how to self-administer in the event that you are not around.

Bronchopulmonary Dysplasia (BPD)

Bronchopulmonary dysplasia (BPD) is a chronic lung disease with persistent difficulty breathing and abnormal changes on the chest X-ray that sometimes follows lung diseases that affect newborn infants. In most cases, BPD occurs after babies have required extra oxygen and/or a mechanical ventilator to treat their original lung problem.

In many cases, the symptoms of BPD disappear quite rapidly. Some infants with BPD may have breathing difficulties for many months or years.

The lungs of an infant with BPD usually contain areas where air sacs have been scarred. This scarring in the lungs that can develop hinders the exchange of oxygen and carbon dioxide between the lung tissue and bloodstream.

Eventually, new lung tissue develops, and the scarred tissue no longer hinders the exchange of oxygen and carbon dioxide. This healing may take months to occur. In the meantime, the infant is dependent on continuous oxygen, may require frequent breathing treatments, and requires special medication and/or percussion postural drainage. Sometimes a cardiopulmonary monitor is required, especially during the first year. This monitor will alarm for any prolonged apnea spells and decreased or increased heart rate.

Babies who are born prematurely or who experience respiratory problems shortly after birth are at risk for bronchopulmonary dysplasia (BPD), sometimes called chronic lung disease. Although most infants fully recover from BPD and have few long-term health problems as a result, BPD can be a serious condition requiring intensive medical care. An infant is not born with BPD. It is something that develops as a consequence of prematurity and progressive lung inflammation.

Bronchopulmonary dysplasia involves abnormal development of lung tissue. It is characterized by inflammation and scarring in the lungs. It develops most often in premature babies who are born with underdeveloped lungs.

Broncho refers to the airways (the bronchial tubes)

through which the oxygen we breathe travels into the lungs. Pulmonary refers to the lungs' tiny air sacs (alveoli) where oxygen and carbon dioxide are exchanged. Dysplasia means abnormal changes in the structure or organization of a group of cells. The cell changes in BPD take place in the smaller airways and lung alveoli, making breathing difficult and causing problems with lung function.

Children with extremely low birth weight (less than 2.2 pounds or 1,000 grams) are most at risk for developing BPD. Although most of these infants eventually outgrow the more serious symptoms, in rare cases, BPD, in combination with other complications of prematurity, can be fatal.

The majority of BPD cases occur in premature infants, usually those who are born at thirty-four weeks' gestation or before and weigh less than 4.5 pounds (2,000 grams). These babies are more likely to be affected by a condition known as infant respiratory distress syndrome (RDS) or hyaline membrane disease, which occurs as a result of tissue damage to the lungs from being on a mechanical ventilator for a significant amount of time.

Mechanical ventilators do the breathing for babies whose lungs are too immature to allow them to breathe on their own. The ventilators also supply necessary oxygen to the lungs of these premature infants. Oxygen is delivered through a tube that has been inserted into the baby's trachea (windpipe) and is given under pressure from the machine to properly move air into stiff, underdeveloped lungs. Sometimes for these babies to survive, the amount of oxygen given must be higher than the oxygen concentration in the air we commonly breathe.

Although mechanical ventilation is essential to their survival, over time the pressure from the ventilation and excess oxygen intake can injure a newborn's delicate lungs, leading to RDS. Almost half of all extremely low birth weight infants will develop some form of RDS. If symptoms of RDS persist, then the condition will be considered BPD if a baby is oxygen dependent at thirty-six weeks postconceptional age. BPD also can arise from other adverse conditions that a newborn's fragile lungs have difficulty coping with, such as trauma, pneumonia, and other infections. All of these can cause the inflammation and scarring associated with BPD, even in a full-term newborn or, very rarely, in older infants and children.

BPD is typically diagnosed if an infant still requires additional oxygen and continues to show signs of respiratory problems after twenty-eight days of age (or past thirty-six weeks postconceptional age). Chest X-rays may be helpful in making the diagnosis. In babies with RDS, the X-rays may show lungs that look like ground glass. In babies with BPD, the X-rays may show lungs that appear spongy.

No available medical treatment can immediately cure bronchopulmonary dysplasia. Treatment is geared to support the breathing and oxygen needs of infants with BPD and to enable them to grow and thrive. Babies first diagnosed with BPD receive intense supportive care in the hospital, usually in a newborn intensive care unit (NICU) until they are able to breathe well enough on their own without the support of a mechanical ventilator.

Infants with BPD are also treated with different kinds of medications that help to support lung function. These include bronchodilators (such as albuterol) to help keep the airways open and diuretics (such as furosemide) to reduce the buildup of fluid in the lungs.

Antibiotics are sometimes needed to fight bacterial infections because babies with BPD are more likely to develop pneumonia. Part of a baby's treatment may involve the administration of surfactant, a natural lubricant that improves breathing function. Babies with RDS who have not yet been diagnosed with BPD may have disrupted surfactant production, so administering natural or synthetic surfactant may reduce the chance that BPD develops.

In addition, babies sick enough to be hospitalized with BPD may need feedings of high-calorie formulas through a gastric tube inserted into the stomach to ensure they get enough calories and nutrients and start to grow.

Improvement for any baby with BPD is gradual. Some infants will be slow to improve; others may not recover from the condition if their lung disease is very severe. Lungs continue to grow for five to seven years, and there can be subtle abnormal lung function even at school age, although the majority of children function well. Many babies diagnosed with BPD will recover close to normal lung function, but this takes time. Scarred, stiffened lung tissue will always have poor function. However, as infants with BPD grow, new healthy lung tissue can form and grow and may eventually take over much of the work of breathing for diseased lung tissue.

Infants with BPD often grow more slowly than other babies and have difficulty gaining weight. They tend to lose weight when they are sick.

As with any child, foster parents have a critical role in the care of an infant with BPD. One important precaution you can take is to reduce the child's exposure to potential respiratory infections. Limit visits from people who are sick, and if the child needs day care, pick a small center where there will be less exposure to infectious agents. Keep the child away from tobacco smoke, particularly in your home, since it is a serious respiratory irritant.

Once a baby comes home from the hospital, foster parents still need to watch for signs of respiratory distress or BPD emergencies, instances in which a child has serious trouble breathing. Signs that an infant might need immediate care include:

- Faster breathing than normal
- Working much harder than usual to breathe
- Belly sinking in with breathing
- Pulling in of the skin between the ribs with each breath
- Growing tired or lethargic from working to breathe
- More coughing than usual
- Panting or grunting
- Wheezing
- Pale, dusky, or blue skin color that may start around the lips or nail beds
- Trouble feeding or excessive spitting up or vomiting of feedings

If you notice any of these symptoms in the child, call the doctor or seek emergency medical attention. Babies with BPD will have different baselines, and you will need to get familiar with the child under your care as soon as possible.

Helpful Tips and Hints for BPD Infant Care:

- Always have an extra oxygen tank full, and oxygen tank keys should be securely attached to the tank.
- Always have an extra nasal cannula for the infant, especially when he or she starts eating baby food. The hardest thing in the world to do is pry carrot, green beans, etc., out of the prongs of the cannula when you are in a hurry.
- Oxygen tanks should be secured while traveling in your car. They should be secured so they cannot roll around in the vehicle.
- When using the cardiopulmonary monitor, it is better to click the electrodes into the wires before placing them on the chest. It can hurt when you press on the chest to make the connection.
- To help keep the infant from getting tangled in the lead wires during sleep at night, it is best to run the wires down sleeper legs and out a hole in the bottom. Another idea is to run the wires down both sides and tape to the side of the diaper.
- Aerosol machines, regardless of make and manufacturer, can mean the difference between a breathing infant and the alternative. Never, for any reason, leave your house to go anywhere unless you have your infant's aerosol machine, medication, dilutent, and mask.

Infantile Apnea

Infantile apnea is when a baby stops breathing for more than twenty seconds or when a baby stops breathing for less than twenty seconds but has other symptoms at the same time such as fainting, pale or blue-colored skin, or a drop in heart rate below eighty.

Some causes of apnea include:

- Infection
- Blocked air passages
- Exposure to drugs in utero
- Congenital heart defects
- Reflux of stomach contents up the esophagus
- Imbalance of body salts
- Convulsions or seizures
- Low blood sugar
- Anemia

Apnea of the premature infant is the most common type of apnea in the newborn. This occurs because the premature infant's brain is still developing and is not completely ready to control the baby's breathing. The apnea stops once the premature baby grows and develops. While the baby is still immature, repeated prolonged apnea may cause low heart rate, fainting, and blueness. These symptoms can lead to low oxygen levels in the blood, possibly causing damage to the baby's vital organs, including the brain. This is why premature babies in the nursery are monitored and treated for apnea with stimulation, medication, or even sometimes with respirator support. The apnea monitor alerts caregivers to apnea before it becomes prolonged so that they may help the baby begin breathing again and avoid symptoms that are more serious.

The reason your baby needs to be on an apnea monitor and the length of the time the monitor is needed depends on the cause of the apnea and how long it has been since any apnea has occurred. The decision to stop using the apnea monitor is a serious one and needs to be made by the baby's physician.

Generally, the monitor is continued until the baby has been apnea free for two months. Siblings of SIDS victims are often monitored until six months of age or two months past the age at which the sibling died. Most premature infants will outgrow the need for a monitor by the time they are three to four months of age.

Respiratory Syncytial Virus (RSV)

RSV stands for respiratory syncytial virus, the most frequent cause of serious respiratory tract infections in infants and children younger than four years of age. This is such a common virus that RSV has infected virtually all children by the age of three. In most young children, it results in a mild respiratory infection that is not distinguishable from a common cold. RSV occurs throughout the year and is most prevalent during the winter months.

RSV causes nasal stuffiness and discharge, cough, and sometimes ear infections. It is usually self-limiting and does not require hospitalization or specific treatment, even in the majority of those who also have lower respiratory tract involvement. These children may have a low-grade fever for several days, respiratory symptoms that may last for one to two weeks, and a cough that sometimes persists beyond two weeks.

Sometimes an infant or young child who is experiencing his or her first RSV infection may develop a severe infection in the lower respiratory tract that is best managed in the hospital. Approximately ninety thousand children are hospitalized with these infections each year. Most commonly, the ones requiring hospitalization are newborns and infants and those who have other complicating or underlying conditions, such as congenital heart disease, lung disease, or prematurity.

A child who develops signs of more stressful breathing, deeper and more frequent coughing, and who generally acts sicker by appearing tired, less playful, and less interested in food may have developed a more serious RSV infection and needs to be hospitalized. In the great majority of cases, RSV infection is self-limiting and requires no specific therapy. For the more serious cases that are hospitalized, the doctor may order an antiviral treatment that is administered in a mist form. This will depend on the severity of the illness, any associated diseases or conditions, and several other factors.

Children and adults of all ages can become infected. The infection in older children and adults may be very mild, usually causing coldlike symptoms. A person becomes infected by coming in close contact with another infected person or with the secretions from an infected person. An infant usually acquires the infection from close contact with an older family member who may have only mild, coldlike symptoms. As noted earlier, RSV occurs throughout the year, but because it occurs in wide-scale, sudden outbreaks, and is so prevalent in the winter months, it is not feasible or advisable to attempt to prevent the normal child's exposure to RSV infection. When a family member is infected, extra precautions may be taken by washing hands often and preventing the spread of infectious secretions on tissues and objects.

Although a child can get a second RSV infection, it is very likely that the symptoms will be much milder than the first time. Most children recover completely and will handle their next respiratory infection with no more difficulty than the average child. A few children, however, appear to be more susceptible to subsequent respiratory problems. Susceptibility may relate, however, to some other underlying medical condition or allergy.

Miscellaneous

Hemangiomas

Hemangiomas are collections of extra blood vessels in the skin and are one of the most common skin problems of the first year of life. Although only 1 to 2.6 percent of newborn infants have hemangiomas present at birth, they are found in up to 10 percent of patients by one year of age and appear most frequently during the first one to four weeks of life. Hemangiomas may have different appearances, depending upon the depth of the increased numbers of blood vessels.

A strawberry hemangioma is an abnormal collection of blood vessels on the skin characterized by a bright red color and well-defined border.

A deep or cavernous hemangioma is a large collection of blood vessels beneath the skin surface characterized by a soft, bluish, or skin-colored mass.

A combined hemangioma is a combination of a deep and superficial (strawberry) hemangioma.

Course of Hemangiomas

Age of child	Hemangiomas
Birth	Often not present or noticeable
1 to 2 months of life	Becomes noticeable
1 to 6 months of life	Grows most rapidly
12 to 18 months of life	Begins to shrink (involute)

Hemangiomas usually involute (shrink away) in time. Thirty percent of hemangiomas will resolve by three years of age, 50 percent by five years of age, and 80 to 90 percent by nine years of age. Over one-half of hemangiomas heal with an excellent cosmetic result without treatment. Hemangiomas in certain areas may have a higher risk of complications. These areas include the face, body folds, and groin.

Hemangiomas in certain locations that affect function

or are complicated by infection or ulceration may be treated with lasers, medications, or injections. Plastic surgery is usually not considered until two to four years of age.

Failure to Thrive

The first few years of life are a time when most children gain weight and grow much more rapidly than they will later on. Sometimes, however, babies and children don't meet expected standards of growth. Although most of these children follow growth patterns that are variations of normal, others are considered to have a failure to thrive.

This is a general diagnosis with many possible causes. Common to all cases, though, is the failure to gain weight as expected, which is often accompanied by poor height growth. Diagnosing and treating a child who fails to thrive focuses on identifying any underlying problem. From there, doctors and the family work together to get the child back into a healthy growth pattern.

Although it's been recognized for more than a century, failure to thrive lacks a precise definition, in part because it describes a condition rather than a specific disease. Children who fail to thrive don't receive or are unable to take in, retain, or utilize the calories needed to gain weight and grow as expected.

Most diagnoses of failure to thrive are made in infants and toddlers in the first few years of life, a crucial period of physical and mental development. After birth, a child's brain grows as much in the first year as it will grow during the rest of the child's life. Poor nutrition during this period can have permanent negative effects on a child's mental development.

Whereas the average term baby doubles his or her birth weight by four months and triples it at one year, children with failure to thrive often don't meet those milestones. Sometimes a child who starts out plump and who shows signs of growing well can begin to fall off in weight gain. After a while, linear (height) growth may slow as well.

If the condition progresses, the undernourished child may:

- Become disinterested in his or her surroundings
- Avoid eye contact
- Become irritable
- Not reach developmental milestones like sitting up, walking, and talking at the usual age

Failure to thrive can result from a wide variety of underlying causes. Some children fail to thrive because of:

- Social factors: In some cases, doctors may not identify a medical problem but may find that the parents are actually causing the failure to thrive. For example, some parents inappropriately restrict the amount of calories they give their infants. They may fear their child will get fat or put him or her on a limited diet similar to one they follow. Or they may simply not feed the child enough either because of a lack of interest or because there are too many distractions in the household, which contributes to the neglect of the child. Living in poverty can also lead to an inability to provide a child with the necessary nutritional requirements.

- Conditions involving the gastrointestinal system like gastroesophageal reflux, chronic diarrhea, cystic fibrosis, chronic liver disease, and celiac disease: With reflux, the esophagus may become so irritated that the child refuses to eat because it hurts. Persistent diarrhea can interfere with the body's ability to hold on to the nutrients and calories from food that's eaten. Cystic fibrosis, chronic liver disease, and celiac disease are conditions that limit the body's ability to absorb nutrients. These are known as malabsorptive disorders. The infant may eat a lot, but his or her body doesn't absorb and retain enough of that food. Celiac disease results from sensitivity to a dietary protein found in wheat and certain other grains. The immune system's abnormal response to this protein causes damage to the lining of the intestine, interfering with its ability to absorb nutrients, a chronic illness or medical disorder.
- Cleft lip: If a child has trouble eating because of prematurity or a cleft lip or palate, for example, he or she may not take in enough calories to support normal growth.
- Cardiac, endocrinologic, and respiratory disorders. These disorders can increase the child's

caloric needs so that it becomes difficult to keep up with them.

- Intolerance of milk protein: This condition can initially lead to difficulty with absorbing nutrients until it's recognized. It can also put an entire class of food out of reach, restricting the child's diet and occasionally leading to failure to thrive.
- Infections (parasites, urinary tract infections, tuberculosis, etc.): These place great energy demands on the body and force it to use nutrients rapidly (and the appetite may be impaired as well), sometimes bringing about short- or long-term failure to thrive.
- Metabolic disorders: These can also limit a child's capacity to make the most of calories consumed. Metabolic disorders might make it difficult for the body to break down, process, or derive energy from food, or they can cause a buildup of toxins during the breakdown process, which can make the child feed poorly or vomit.

In some cases, doctors are unable to pinpoint a specific cause.

Although doctors in the past tended to categorize cases of failure to thrive as either organic (caused by an underlying medical disorder) or inorganic (caused by caregivers' or parents' actions), they're less likely to make such sharp distinctions today. That's because medical and behavioral causes often appear together.

For instance, if a baby has severe reflux and is reluctant to eat, feeding times can be stressful for a caregiver. He or she may become tense and frustrated, and this may make it difficult for the caregiver to sustain attempts to feed the child adequate amounts of food.

Many normal babies go through brief periods when their weight gain plateaus or they even lose a little weight. However, if a baby doesn't gain weight for three consecutive months during the first year of life, doctors usually become concerned.

Doctors diagnose failure to thrive by using standard growth charts to plot the child's weight, length, and head circumference, which are measured at each well-baby exam. Children who fall below a certain weight range for their age or who are failing to gain weight at the expected rate will likely be evaluated further to determine if there is a problem.

Along with obtaining a thorough medical and feeding history and performing a detailed physical examination, the doctor may order a complete blood count, urinalysis, and various blood chemical and electrolyte tests that can be helpful in the search for underlying medical problems. If the doctor suspects a particular disease or disorder as a possible cause, he or she may perform additional specific tests to identify that condition.

To determine whether the child is receiving enough food, the child's doctor (sometimes with the help of a dietitian) will do a calorie count after asking the parents what the child eats every day. And talking to the parents can help a doctor identify any problems at home, such as neglect, poverty, household stress, or feeding difficulties.

Children with failure to thrive need the help of their

parents and a doctor. Sometimes an entire medical team will work on the child's case.

In addition to the child's primary doctor, the team might include a nutritionist to evaluate the child's dietary needs and an occupational or speech therapist to help the caregiver and child develop successful feeding behaviors and address any sucking or swallowing problems the child might have. Occupational and speech therapists are often helpful because of their expertise in the muscular control that's involved in eating.

Because treatment of failure to thrive involves treating any disease or disorder causing the problem, specialists such as a cardiologist, neurologist, or gastroenterologist may also be part of the care team.

Particularly in cases of failure to thrive that are thought to be caused by caregivers' or parents' actions, a social worker and a psychologist or other mental health professional may help address problems in the child's home environment and provide any needed support.

Often, in cases of poor nutrition, the treatment can be carried out at home with frequent follow-up visits to the doctor's office or clinic. The doctor will recommend high-calorie foods and place an infant on a high-calorie formula.

More severe cases may call for tube feedings in which a tube is put in that runs from the nose into the stomach. Liquid nutrition is provided at a steady rate through the tube. Once the tube is put in place, the child is usually fed at night, so as not to interfere with his or her activities or limit the child's desire to eat during the day. (About half of a child's caloric needs can be delivered at night through a continuous drip.) Once the child is more adequately nourished, he or she will feel better and will probably start to eat more on his or her own. At that point, the tube can be removed.

A child with extreme failure to thrive may need to be hospitalized so that he or she can be fed and monitored continuously. During this time, any possible underlying causes of the condition can be evaluated and treated appropriately. This also gives the treatment team the opportunity to observe firsthand the caregiver's feeding technique and the interaction between caregiver and child during feedings and at other times.

How long treatment lasts varies significantly from case to case. Weight gain takes time, so several months may pass before a child is back in the normal range for his or her age. Children who require hospitalization may stay for ten to fourteen days or more to establish satisfactory weight gain, but it can be many months until the symptoms of severe malnutrition are no longer present. Failure to thrive caused by a chronic illness or disorder may have to be monitored periodically and treated for even longer, perhaps for a lifetime.

If you're worried that the child under your care is failing to thrive, remember that there are many reasons why he or she might be slower to gain weight other than failure to thrive. For instance, breastfed babies and bottle-fed babies often gain weight at different rates in the early newborn period.

As a guideline, babies usually eat eight to twelve times in a twenty-four-hour period (a couple of ounces [sixty milliliters] every few hours) in the first weeks after birth.

By the time they're two to three months old, the number of feedings has dropped to six to eight, but the amount they eat each time has increased. At four months, about thirty ounces (890 milliliters) a day provides sufficient nutrition for most bottle-fed infants.

The child's doctor will have plenty of opportunities to identify a problem at regular well-baby checkups. You can also periodically check the baby's weight at home if you feel you need the reassurance.

If you notice a drop in weight gain or the baby doesn't seem to have a normal appetite, get in touch with the child's doctor. Any major change in eating pattern also warrants a call to the doctor. Toddlers and other kids may have days and sometimes weeks when they show little interest in eating, but that shouldn't happen in infants.

Hernias

A hernia is a loop of bowel from the abdomen that goes into an area where it normally would not be. In babies the most common hernias are inguinal hernias and umbilical hernias. An inguinal hernia develops in the groin at the level of the skin crease between the leg and the abdomen. In a baby boy the bowel loop goes into the scrotum. An umbilical hernia develops after the cord comes off and is an outpouching where the cord used to be. Hernias are usually not present when the baby is born but develop later.

A hernia develops when there is a failure of certain openings to close during development. Normally the sides of these tissues come together and then seal over. If they don't seal, they can reopen and then fluid and loops of bowel can slide into the opening or sac. The closing process usually occurs in utero when the baby's tummy is flat and the intestines are small. When babies are born prematurely and they use their intestines earlier, there is more pressure and fullness to the tummy. This makes the risk for a hernia greater.

Hernias are more common in smaller babies, baby boys, and babies who have had lung disease.

Umbilical hernias will usually go away during the first year or two of life. They only need to be repaired surgically if they become very large or if a loop of bowel gets caught or trapped in the hernia (incarcerated). Inguinal hernias usually need to be repaired surgically. The timing of surgery varies.

When a loop of bowel gets caught in the hernia, it swells. This cuts off the blood supply to that loop of bowel, and the bowel loop can die and/or rupture. Also, in a boy baby, the swollen loop of bowel can cut off the blood supply to the testicle on the hernia side, causing injury or death to the testicle. Incarceration is a rare event.

There are several signs of incarceration. Not all may be present. These include inconsolable crying, pain, soreness or tenderness over the hernia, redness or bluish color in the groin or scrotum, and/or vomiting.

Kidney Diseases in Childhood

The kidneys play a critical role in the body. Acting as the body's filtering system, they help control water levels and eliminate wastes through urine. They also help regulate blood pressure, red blood cell production, and the levels of calcium and minerals.

But sometimes the kidneys don't develop properly and as a result, don't function the way that they should. Often these problems are genetic and not due to anything a parent did or didn't do.

Many of these problems can be diagnosed before a baby is born through routine prenatal testing and treated with medication or surgery while the child is still young. Other problems may emerge later, such as symptoms of urinary infections, growth retardation, high blood pressure, etc. In some cases, the problems are more severe and require more extensive surgical treatment.

The kidneys are like the body's garbage collection and disposal system. Through microscopic units called nephrons, the kidneys remove waste products and extra water from the food a person eats, returning chemicals the body needs (such as sodium, phosphorus, and potassium) back into the bloodstream. The extra water combines with other waste to become urine, which flows through thin tubes called ureters to the bladder, where it stays until it exits through the urethra (the tube that carries urine out of the body from the bladder) when someone goes to the bathroom.

The kidneys also produce three important hormones: erythropoietin, which stimulates the bone marrow to make red blood cells; renin, which helps regulate blood pressure; and the active form of vitamin D, which helps control the calcium balance in the body and maintain healthy bones.

Kidney failure, which is also called renal failure, is

when the kidneys slow down or stop properly filtering wastes from the body, which can cause buildups of waste products and toxic substances in the blood. Kidney failure can be acute (which means sudden) or chronic (occurring over time and usually long lasting or permanent).

Acute kidney failure may be due to bacterial infection, injury, shock, heart failure, poisoning, or drug overdose. Treatment includes correcting the problem that led to the failure and in rare cases requires dialysis.

Chronic kidney failure involves a deterioration of kidney function over time. In kids and teens, it can result from acute kidney failure that fails to improve, birth defects, chronic kidney diseases, or chronic severe high blood pressure. If diagnosed early, chronic kidney failure can be treated. The goal of treatment usually is to slow the decline of kidney function with medication, blood pressure control, and diet. At some point, a kidney transplant may be required.

The most common kidney diseases in children are present at birth. They include:

- Posterior urethral valve obstruction: This narrowing or obstruction of the urethra affects only boys. It can be diagnosed before the baby is born or just afterward and treated with surgery.
- Fetal hydronephrosis: This enlargement of one or both of the kidneys is caused by either an obstruction in the developing urinary tract or a condition called vesicoureteral reflux (VUR) in which urine abnormally flows backward (or refluxes) from the bladder into the ureters. Fetal

hydronephrosis is usually diagnosed before the child is born and treatment varies widely. In some cases the condition only requires ongoing monitoring; in others, surgery must be done to clear the obstruction from the urinary tract.

- Polycystic kidney disease (PKD): This is a condition in which many fluidfilled cysts develop in both kidneys. The cysts can multiply so much and grow so large that they lead to kidney failure. Most forms of PKD are inherited. Doctors can diagnose the condition before or after the child is born. In some cases there are no symptoms; in others, PKD can lead to urinary tract infections, kidney stones, and high blood pressure. Treatment for PKD also varies widely. In some cases, PKD can be managed with dietary changes; in others, it requires a kidney transplant or dialysis, which is a medical treatment that helps the body filter waste when the kidneys can't do the job.
- Multicystic kidney disease: This is when large cysts develop in a kidney that hasn't developed properly, eventually causing it to stop functioning. (While PKD always affects both kidneys, multicystic kidney disease usually affects only one kidney.) Usually diagnosed before a baby is born, this condition can lead to kidney failure. Currently, there is no cure, but doctors can manage it by preventing and treating infections, maintaining blood pressure, and addressing any issues that arise with surgery.
- Renal tubular acidosis: This is a condition in

which the kidneys do not properly regulate the amount of acid in the body. It can cause kidney stones and affect a child's growth but usually can be treated with medications.

- Wilms tumor: This is a type of childhood cancer that involves the kidney. It is typically diagnosed within the first two years of life and can be treated with surgery and chemotherapy.
- Glomerulonephritis: This is an inflammation or infection of the glomeruli, which are parts of the nephrons that contain tiny blood vessels. It can affect the kidney's ability to properly filter out waste and can lead to swelling, blood in the urine, and a reduced amount of urine production. Some cases can be treated with medication while others require dialysis or a kidney transplant.
- Nephrotic syndrome: This occurs when the body loses large amounts of protein through the urine, typically because of some sort of change in the nephrons. It is usually diagnosed after the child is one year old. Swelling of the face, abdomen, and extremities are among the main symptoms and are often relieved with medication.

As a child develops in the womb, a part of the urinary tract can grow to an abnormal size or in an abnormal shape or position. These problems include:

- Duplication of the ureters: kidney has two ureters instead of one. This can lead to urinary tract infections over time and can be treated with medication or occasionally with surgery.

- Horseshoe kidney: where the two kidneys are fused (connected) into one arched kidney that usually functions normally, but is more prone to develop problems later in life. An uncomplicated horseshoe kidney does not need medical or surgical treatment, but it does need to be checked regularly by doctors.

Sometimes a child can have other health problems that affect how well the kidneys function. These can include:

- High blood pressure or hypertension: The kidneys control blood pressure by regulating the amount of salt in the body and by making the enzyme renin that, along with other substances, controls the constriction of blood vessels. The many causes of high blood pressure include any of the kidney diseases mentioned above, genetic factors such as the so-called essential hypertension, which is the most common form of high blood pressure in adults, and obesity, which has become a major factor.
- Kidney stones: The result of the build-up of crystallized salts and minerals such as calcium in the urinary tract, kidney stones (also called calculi) also can form after an infection. If kidney stones are large enough to block the kidney or ureter, they can cause severe abdominal pain. But the stones usually pass through the urinary tract on their own. In some cases, they need to

be removed surgically or treated with medication or modifications to the diet. Sometimes the first symptoms are pain and blood in the urine. Kidney stones are more common in adults than they are in kids.

- Nephritis: This is any inflammation of the kidney. It can be caused by infection, an autoimmune disease (such as lupus), or an unknown reason. The first symptoms of nephritis usually are high levels of protein and blood in the urine.
- Urinary tract infections (UTI): UTIs are typically caused by bacteria, such as E. coli. Most UTIs occur in the lower urinary tract, in the bladder and urethra, and they can cause pain during urination and a fever. Treatment with antibiotics should be started as soon as possible so the infection doesn't spread to the kidneys, where it can cause irreversible damage. In babies, UTIs tend to be more common in boys than girls, perhaps because boys are more affected by congenital kidney problems that predispose them to infection. Later in life, girls are more likely to get UTIs because of their shorter urethras. Bad habits can contribute to UTIs—kids holding it when they need to go to the bathroom or wiping themselves in the wrong direction after using the toilet (they should wipe from front to back so bacteria from the stool do not get into the urethra). Among teens, girls are more likely to develop UTIs than boys, mostly due to the shorter urethra or sexual activity with a full bladder.

The signs and symptoms of urinary tract or kidney problems are diverse and include:

- Fever
- Swelling around the eyes, face, feet, and ankles (also known as edema)
- Burning or pain during urination
- Significant increase in the frequency of urination
- Difficulty in controlling urination in children who are mature enough to use the toilet
- Recurrence of nighttime bedwetting (in children who have been dry for several months)
- Blood in the urine
- High blood pressure

If the child's doctor suspects a kidney disease in the child, he or she will likely take a medical history, do a physical exam, and order urine tests, blood tests, imaging studies, or a biopsy to help make a diagnosis. These studies are usually suggested by a nephrologist, a doctor who specializes in the diagnosis and treatment of kidney diseases.

With urinalysis (a type of urine test), the child's doctor can quickly detect abnormalities (such as too many red blood cells) that may signal inflammation or irritation in the urinary tract. Urinalysis can also detect excess white blood cells, which is most commonly associated with bladder and kidney infections.

Certain blood tests tell doctors how well the kidneys

are filtering waste products and balancing the bloodstream's chemical makeup.

Two other important diagnostic tools a doctor may use are blood pressure and growth measurements. Along with the heart, the kidneys are crucial to determining blood pressure. High blood pressure in a child is an important sign that the kidneys need to be evaluated. Accurate growth measurements can provide a clue to diagnosing some kidney diseases because children with chronic kidney disease often grow poorly.

The child's doctor may use a kidney biopsy to evaluate the child's kidney function. A biopsy is a procedure in which a small piece of the kidney tissue is removed with a needle. Performed while a child is under anesthesia, it's a simple procedure that can help make an accurate diagnosis of the kidney problem in about nine out of ten cases. It's especially helpful in the diagnosis of nephritis and nephrosis.

The doctor also will take a medical history by asking you about any concerns and symptoms, the child's past health, family's health, past medications, any allergies, and other issues.

In addition to standard X-rays, other imaging studies a doctor may use to help diagnose kidney diseases include:

- Ultrasound: A renal ultrasound shows details of the anatomy of the kidneys and bladder. It can rule out or diagnose obstructions, developmental abnormalities, tumors, and stones in the kidneys and urinary tract.

- Computerized tomography (CT): It can show if the kidneys have developed properly or if the flow of urine is blocked by a stone or a developmental abnormality.
- Renal nuclear scan: The scan shows how the kidneys compare to each other in size, shape, and function. It also can detect scarring or other evidence of recurrent or chronic kidney infection.
- Voiding cystourethrogram (VCUG): VCUG is commonly used to evaluate the bladder and the ureters. This procedure involves putting a dye into the bladder to see whether there's an obstruction or VUR when the child urinates.

Treatment begins with diet modification and medicines. The child may need to take several medicines, including vitamins, calcium, bicarbonate, and blood pressure pills. As a result, medication management may be a major challenge.

Children with chronic kidney failure may not have any symptoms until about 80 percent of their kidney function is lost. Then they may feel tired, have nausea or vomiting, have difficulty concentrating, or experience confusion. Accumulated fluid appears as swelling in the skin, fluid congestion in the lungs, and high blood pressure. At this stage, two treatment options are available: dialysis and transplant.

Nearly all children with end-stage kidney disease eventually receive transplants. If a living related donor can't be found, dialysis may be required until a donor kidney is found.

Retinopathy of Prematurity

Retinopathy of prematurity is a bilateral disease of the retinal vessels present in premature infants, some of whom were exposed to high postnatal oxygen concentrations. High oxygen concentration used in treating premature infants, especially those weighing less than 1,500 grams causes vasoconstriction of the immature retinal vessels and eventually occlusion of the vessels. Fibrous proliferation and invasion of the vitreous may follow this. Retinal detachment may occur at that time or many years later. Blindness develops within several weeks. Other factors can give an important role in the pathogenesis of retinopathy of prematurity (ROP). Apnea, asphyxia, sepsis, nutritional deficiencies, and a large number of blood transfusions given over a short period of time have all been connected to ROP.

Prevention is possible by using only the lowest possible effective oxygen concentration in treating premature infants. Thus, the lowest level possible without endangering the life of the infant is used. Too severe restriction of oxygen will increase the likelihood of hyaline membrane disease and neurologic disorders. All premature infants treated with supplemental oxygen should have a careful examination by an ophthalmologist prior to discharge from the hospital. Once blindness develops, there is no effective treatment.

Tracheomalacia

Tracheomalacia is a weakness and floppiness of the walls of the trachea (main airway). There are three types of tracheomalacia. One type is congenital (present at birth); the others are acquired, meaning that the trachea is normal at birth but becomes floppy later in life.

Tracheomalacia in a newborn occurs when the cartilage in the trachea has not developed properly. This causes the wall of the trachea to be floppy rather than relatively rigid, as it is supposed to be. Breathing difficulties associated with congenital tracheomalacia (also called type 1) begin soon after birth.

Other types of tracheomalacia occur due to degeneration of previously normal cartilage in the wall of the trachea. This can happen when something outside the trachea causes pressure on the airway (for example, an abnormality of the blood vessels surrounding the trachea or a tumor in the neck or throat). This is called type 2 tracheomalacia. Breakdown of the cartilage in the trachea can also result from prolonged intubation or chronic infections involving the trachea. This is called type 3 tracheomalacia.

All three types of tracheomalacia are very uncommon. Common symptoms are:

- High-pitched breathing (stridor) and rattling, noisy breaths
- Breathing problems that get worse with coughing, crying, feeding (in the case of infants) or upper respiratory infections
- Breathing noises that may change with position and improve during sleep

A doctor's examination confirms the symptoms. A chest X-ray may show narrowing of the trachea when exhaling. Even if the X-ray is normal, it is needed to rule out other problems.

A definitive diagnosis is obtained by laryngoscopy, which is performed by an otolaryngologist (ear, nose, and throat doctor, or ENT). This allows the airway anatomy to be seen and helps determine the extent of tracheomalacia.

Infants with tracheomalacia must be monitored closely when they have respiratory infections. Most infants respond well to humidified air, physical therapy, careful feedings, and antibiotics for infections.

Congenital tracheomalacia generally resolves on its own by the age of eighteen to twenty-four months. As the tracheal cartilage strengthens and the trachea grows, the noisy respirations and breathing difficulties gradually stop.

Babies born with tracheomalacia may have other congenital abnormalities, such as heart defects, developmental delay, or gastroesophageal reflux.

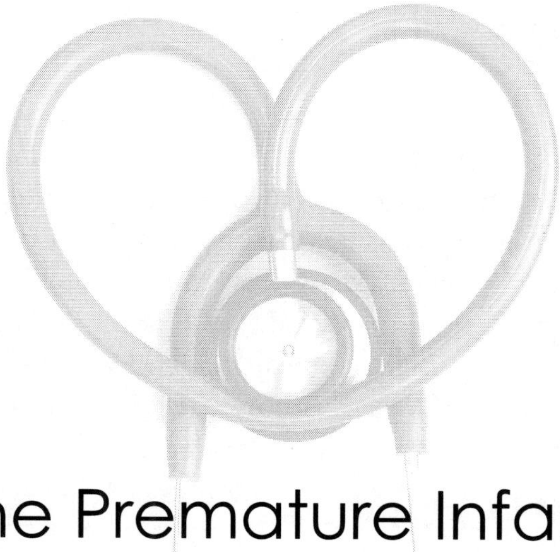

The Premature Infant

We are going to talk about the premature infant and interventions to help the drug-exposed infant in this chapter. Frequently, infants in your care that are premature have been drug exposed with little or no prenatal care. These infants can be very challenging but will improve with calm, loving care.

Behaviors of the Drug- and/ or Alcohol-Exposed Infants

Infants who have been prenatally exposed to drugs and/or alcohol often have unique care needs. This information has been developed to help you better understand the infant and how to care for these special babies. Other infants may have none or very few of these problems. They are all different. Each one has been exposed to drugs and/or alcohol to a different degree and at different times of development. Exposure to drugs in utero can cause infants' states to vary from highly irritable to very passive. Most drug-exposed infants are highly irritable and have difficulty sleeping, and irritable infants can reach a frantic crying state very quickly. Some infants who have been prenatally exposed to drugs and/or alcohol will act in the following manner:

- Irritable
- Jitteriness or tremors
- Stiff muscles (hypertonia)
- Frantic sucking
- Poor feeding
- Staring or unusual eye movements
- Poor eye contact
- Diarrhea
- Fitful cry, high-pitched cry
- Crying for prolonged periods of time
- Unusual drowsiness or sleepiness
- Unusually short periods of sleep

Stiffness and rigidity are increased extensor tone and are often seen in infants prenatally exposed to drugs or alcohol. They have increased muscle tone and will frequently roll over at a very early age. Because of the stiffness, they do not have the ability to cuddle and will remain stiff when being held. They will also tend to arch their backs.

This occurs up to twelve months of age. Warm baths and massage can sometimes help relax the infant. In addition, placing the infant in a cloth sling on the hip will help decrease abnormal extension pattern, decrease irritability, and increase tolerance of touch.

Feeding time is important for all babies. Infants exposed prenatally to drugs and/or alcohol may have some special needs in this area. The following are some tips you may find helpful for making feedings more satisfying:

- Swaddle baby snugly during feedings.
- Be very calm and use slow, quiet care.
- It is best if they have only one caretaker to begin with.
- Talk softly to them but do not expose them to excess noise or activity.
- You may have to use a preemie nipple and enlarge the hole with a sterile needle because the baby will tire easily. They often do not suck effectively and need time to get the hang of it.

Calming Interventions:

- Avoid quick movements in picking up infant
- Baby may require a lot of holding
- Carry or rock in vertical position
- Cuddling
- Slow rocking
- Singing, soft talking

- Swaddling with blanket
- Pacifier
- Bottle with formula warmed
- Gentle interaction (low-key stimulation)
- Swing
- Music tape with lullabies and heartbeat
- Warm baths

The main secret is to handle baby slowly, frequently, calmly, and with warmth and gentleness to avoid reaching a frantic state.

Tremors of the hands, arms, legs, chin, and tongue are commonly observed in infants exposed to drugs in utero. These are very common in newborn infants but can be seen in older children up to one year. Tremors are seen while the infant is at rest and will be noticed more when the infant is extremely tired. As they grow older, the tremors become less intense and tend to diminish. Tremors will become more intense if the infant is trying to reach for objects or attempting a specific motor skill.

Infants with special needs can be difficult to care for. Remember that there is only so much you can do. You need to take care of yourself too. It may be necessary to let the baby cry. This is sometimes appropriate when all interventions fail and you need a timeout. Place the baby in a safe environment and do something to relax. The baby will be safe, and this time will allow you to provide better care to this challenging child. It is very important to have alternate caregivers. They also need to be trained on the challenges of caring for these children and calming interventions. Remember, as the child grows and is able to handle different situations, you will be rewarded for your hard work with a baby who calms and can be comforted.

Interventions to Decrease Stress in the Drug-Exposed Infant

- Decrease lights and noise in room, including TV/radio.
- Wrap the baby snugly with hands midline. This helps to overcome extensor tone.
- Always place baby on back or side to sleep, never on tummy.
- Hold the baby's hands midline over the baby's chest with one of your hands, exerting a secure feeling.
- Try rocking with baby held vertically. This is often more successful than horizontal rocking.
- Frequent warm-water baths help calm them.
- If baby is averting your gaze, it is likely due to overstimulation by simple eye contact with you. Sit the baby on your lap, snugly wrapped, facing away from you.
- Do not use walkers with these infants. Walkers increase predisposition to weight to bear on toes.
- Protect the baby's knees from irritation during periods of frantic fussiness.
- Use a pacifier to help with their non-nutritive sucking needs.

Growth and Development: Premature Infant: Feeding and Weight Gain

Studies have shown that most preemies do as well as other children once they have had a few months to catch up. Babies who were very tiny (twenty-four to twenty-eight weeks) and babies who were very sick or who still have many medical problems when they go home often have a longer period of catch-up growth. Routine exams are done to be sure the baby's mental and physical development are okay and that he can do all the things he is supposed to do at his age.

- All babies are different. However, the sicker and smaller the baby, the more differences you will see for a while.
- A premature infant may have a softer cry for shorter periods of time.
- A premature infant may have jerky, jittery movements.
- The premature baby has ways of telling you when he is overtired, stressed, or needs a break. He may yawn, stretch, spit up, breathe faster, become pale or mottled in color, become limp, close his eyes, look away, arch his back, or stiffen his arms or legs. These are called timeout signs.

A preemie baby actually has two birthdays: the day he was born and the day he was expected to be born. Adjusted age is a better yardstick for measuring a preemie's progress as it counts the baby's age from the time he should have been born, not the time he was really born.

For example, Sarah was born on September 17, two months before she was due, so we can start counting her adjusted age from the time of her due date on November 17. By December 17, Sarah's real age is three months, but her adjusted age is one month.

Feeding a premature baby may be different from feeding a term baby. Prematurity often alters the development of normal healthy eating patterns. Feeding can be exhausting and require a lot of energy for a preemie. This can be related to how sick he was while in the hospital and how early he was born. Some premature infants who were intubated for a long period of time may have negative responses to anything in their mouths. A premature infant can also have poor control of suck, swallow, and breathing patterns due to an immature central nervous system. Consequently, nippling can lead to abnormal feeding patterns, exhaustion, and breathing difficulties.

The following are some guidelines that may be helpful in feeding a premature infant:

- The preemie may wake up and want to eat every two to three hours, or he may be sleepy during the feeding, or he may set his own schedule, waking thirty minutes to an hour before feeding.
- If the baby is not awake when a feeding is due, wake him up by changing his position or loosening the covers. He will be more successful at feeding if he is brought to a more alert state.

- Feed the baby in a quiet environment, preferably with indirect lighting.
- Coordinate baby's suck and swallow with his respirations to allow him adequate breathing time.
- Allow the baby to set the pace for the feeding. Preterm infants may require more time to complete a feeding than term infants.
- Do not push the feeding beyond the baby's capabilities.
- Premature infants tend to spit up more than term newborns. The valve, or opening, between the esophagus and stomach is not tight, so he may tend to spit up small amounts with feeding and burping.

Weight Gain and Growth for Premature Infants

- A healthy premature baby who is eating well and who was the right size for the time he was born can be expected to grow at the same rate as a full-term baby of the same corrected age.
- Normal size for age is usually reached at about ten months after the time the baby should have been born.
- The very ill premature baby born with the appropriate weight may have very rapid catch-up growth at six to nine months corrected age. If the growth continues, his size will continue to increase. If the growth slows, the child may remain small.

- A baby born small for his gestational age may tend to remain small during childhood.
- The preschool child who was a very low-birth-weight baby (less than 1,500 grams or three and a half pounds) may tend to be slender, although normal height.

Nutritional Needs of the Premature Infant

Nutritional needs for premature infants are very special and important. Their bodies are often working twice as hard to maintain a healthy balance and will require more nutrients than a nonfragile infant. If they do not receive the necessary amount of nutrition, they will fail to thrive (poor weight gain), be more prone to infections, and their development can often be delayed. Besides having an increase of nutritional needs, many premature infants will have feeding problems related to being premature or illnesses affecting the digestive system.

The following are the most common situations that may require special care after discharge.

Poor Suck/Swallow

The ability to suck, swallow, and breathe is a very synchronized skill organized by the brain. Premature infants, depending on the extent of prematurely, have trouble coordinating their suck, swallow, and breathing. They are most often fed by gavage until their coordination improves. If the infant has experienced any neurological complications, the poor suck/swallow may persist for a longer period, and gavage feedings may need to continue in the home. Often, if the condition appears to be long term, a gastrostomy tube is surgically placed to make feedings simple and less risky for damage to the back of the throat.

GE Reflux (GI Reflux)

GE reflux is the result of poor muscle tone in the muscle sphincter (esophageal sphincter) at the top of the stomach. When the muscle tone is poor, the formula can easily flow back up the esophagus. If the reflux is severe, there is a risk of aspiration (into the lungs) and apnea/bradycardia. The most common treatment is thickening of the formula and elevation of the head after feedings. If severe, a medication is used, along with a home monitor for apnea and bradycardia.

Necrotizing Enterocolitis (NEC)

NEC is a condition that can occur in very low-birth-weight infants who have been very stressed. The exact cause is still unclear, but bacteria will invade the tissue walls of the intestine. The bacteria forms gas bubbles that cause swelling, which interferes with the blood flow to that area of the intestine. If severe, intestinal tissue will die and break open, spreading infection through the abdominal cavity. If this occurs, surgery is necessary to remove the dead intestinal tissue. Sometimes a large section of the intestine must be removed and the intestine cannot be reconnected; then an ileostomy or colostomy is constructed. The ileostomy or colostomy connects the intestine to the outside of the abdomen where a drainage bag is attached to receive the intestinal contents. Usually six to twelve months later, surgery may be attempted to reconnect the intestine.

Short Bowel Syndrome

This condition is a result of necessary surgical removal of a large part of the intestine, most often because of NEC. The intestinal contents move through the intestine very rapidly, and the time to reabsorb the fluid and salts is decreased. The result is diarrhea-type stools, loss of necessary body salts, and poor absorption of nutrients. Often, a special predigested formula is necessary for quick absorption and dietary replacement of salts (NaCL, KCL) and vitamins. Skin care is another major concern; frequent watery stools can quickly cause the skin to break down. Special diaper care and ointments are necessary, such as Bag Balm, Desitin, etc.

The Sick Premature Infant

Many premature infants are resilient and surprise everyone by overcoming great odds. But premature infants are also vulnerable to infection and to complications related to immature body organs. With each additional week of prematurity, a newborn is at greater risk of having medical problems. Infants who have reached their thirty-second week of development before birth are considered less at risk for complications than those who are born earlier. The most common complications of prematurity result from immature organs and an immature immune system and include:

- Low blood pressure
- Low blood sugar
- Anemia
- Respiratory distress syndrome
- Chronic lung disease (also known as bronchopulmonary dysplasia)
- Necrotizing enterocolitis
- Patent ductus arteriosus
- Infection (including sepsis)
- Retinopathy of prematurity
- Intraventricular hemorrhage, or bleeding in the brain, which can result in cerebral palsy or mental retardation
- Inguinal hernia

Any infant born before term (before thirty-seven completed weeks gestation) has an increased risk of developing medical complications. Infants born at thirty-two weeks gestation or older are least likely to develop complications. With each additional week of prematurity before thirty-two weeks, risks begin to increase dramatically. Infants born at twenty-three to twenty-six weeks gestation are extremely underdeveloped and have a significantly higher risk of death and disability. Parents of these infants are likely to be faced with difficult life-or-death medical decisions.

Before you take the baby home, you will want to:

- Discuss any questions and concerns with the neonatal intensive care unit (NICU) staff and the baby's doctor.
- Make a pediatric appointment for a few days after the infant's homecoming. Weekly medical checks after discharge are especially important for a premature infant.
- If home-based health care and supportive therapies are available to you, take advantage of them. Home-based services spare you and the infant the physical and emotional stress of traveling to numerous appointments.

Medical problems associated with prematurity are frequently complex, and a multidisciplinary approach is often required. Some common problems include the following:

- Anemia, which can be reduced by iron supplementation
- Cerebral palsy or mental retardation as a result of intraventricular hemorrhage or periventricular leukomalacia
- Respiratory problems, including bronchopulmonary dysplasia and apnea
- Visual problems, such as those associated with retinopathy of prematurity

- Gastroesophageal reflux
- Surgical problems, including inguinal or umbilical hernia and cryptorchidism

Monitoring of growth and development includes recording the infant's head circumference, weight, and length on a growth chart for premature infants. Nutritional status should be assessed at each visit, watching for hyperosmolar problems in infants receiving high-calorie formulas. Consultation with other specialists may be required if abnormalities are identified during follow-up care in the office.

Advancements in the care of premature infants have led to increased survival of these infants, and family physicians frequently provide care to these infants following their discharge from the hospital. Premature infants present many challenges to the family physician. Medical problems originating in the initial weeks of life may require care for months or years. Other conditions may manifest clinically later in infancy or in childhood, necessitating an attitude of continual alertness and attentiveness on the part of the physician.

Abnormalities found in screening frequently require consultation with other specialists. Coordination of health care for timely intervention and follow-up is an important role for the family physician.

Anemia is common but can be minimized by using iron supplements. Careful physical examinations and monitoring of developmental milestones help identify cerebral palsy or other developmental abnormalities. The presence of developmental abnormalities signals the need for multidisciplinary evaluation. Chronic medical problems can be managed by the family physician, along with the neonatologist. Surgical referral for hernias and cryptorchidism must be obtained in a timely fashion. By performing frequent examinations, coordinating the infant's medical care, and monitoring the needs of the parents, the family physician can make effective interventions on behalf of the premature infant.

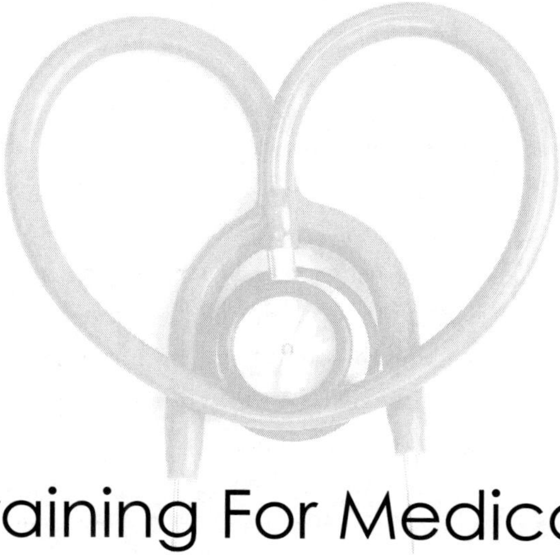

Training For Medical Procedures: How to Get It

You are responsible for getting all the necessary medical training for the medically fragile child you will be caring for. There are many resources that are available to you, such as the registered nurse (i.e., public health nurse or the registered nurse covering your home), the bedside nurse who has been taking care of the child at the hospital, or the specially trained nurses on staff at the hospital. Some examples are the ostomy nurse, TPN nurse, wound care nurse, or other specially trained nurses. You also have available the other licensed staff, such as the respiratory therapist, physical therapist, or occupational therapist, to name a few.

It may be necessary to make appointments with the staff. This will ensure that you get all your questions answered and the care is explained thoroughly. Before you take this medically fragile child home, you need to make sure that you are comfortable with all the care this child may need. Don't be pressured into taking this child home until you are comfortable. Remember, you will be the one at home responsible for the care. Ask any question about the care involved, no matter how silly it may seem to you. Remember, it is okay to speak up! And if you feel you are not getting the information you need, ask to speak with a supervisor.

The nurse case manager is responsible for ordering medical supplies for the baby prior to discharge. Usually they will have a relationship with a vendor and all the equipment will be delivered and explained to you before you take the baby home. Information on how to order, how often, and contact personnel will all be explained. Again, if it is not clear or you don't understand, don't hesitate to ask.

It is a good idea to arrive at your training sessions with a training checklist. (See sample, more in index) This will provide a guideline for your questions, and by also using the checklist and having the licensed staff that is training you sign it, you are providing the necessary documentation for licensing. You are required to have training for each individual child. Even if you have another child (or had) with the same diagnosis, you are still required to receive medical training for that individual child.

You may be exempted by the child's individualized health care team from all or part of the training requirements if you are a health care professional and training is determined to be unnecessary based upon your professional qualifications and expertise.

I have provided a few samples of training checklists. You can easily make a list using the medical conditions the child has and the medical procedures that are required. Take your list to the training sessions and have the health care professional review it and sign. Most babies will have a combination of needs, and you may need to have training with more than one health care professional.

Training Checklist for Cardiac Disease and G-Tube

_____ Reviewed all medications, dosage, frequency and possible side effects.

_____ Instructed on clinical manifestations and pathophysiology of heart and lung condition.

_____ Instructed on S/S of increased oxygen requirements, and respiratory distress. Interventions discussed such as oxygen via mask or nasal cannula, calming baby and/or calling 911.

_____ Instructed with return demonstration of mixing of proper formula, frequency, and maintenance. Discussed feeding goals, feeding schedule, and techniques.

_____ Instructed with return demonstration on GT site cleaning, and S/S of site infection.

_____ Instructed with return demonstration on GT feedings, frequency, medication administration, and adverse effects of GT feedings.

Signature/Title of Person Trained: ____________________
Date: ________

Signature/Title of Trainer: __________________________
Date: ________

Training Checklist for the Premature Infant

_____ State the S/S of apnea and bradycardia of prematurely.

_____ Reviewed with demonstration all medications, dosage, frequency and possible side effects.

_____ Discussed feeding goals, feeding schedule, and techniques.

_____ Instructed on S/S of increased oxygen requirements, and respiratory distress. Interventions discussed such as 911 or medical care.

_____ Discussed growth and development for the premature infant and adjusted age development.

Signature/Title of Person Trained: ____________________
Date: ________

Signature/Title of Trainer:_________________________
Date: ________

Training Checklist for Bronchopulmonary Dysplasia

_____ Reviewed the pathophysiology of bronchopulmonary dysplasia and state the S/S of respiratory distress.

_____ State the S/S of apnea and bradycardia of prematurely.

_____ Reviewed with demonstration all medications, dosage, frequency and possible side effects.

_____ Instructed and returned demonstration on the use of apnea monitor, how to respond to an alarm, assess the situation, and possible interventions.

_____ Instructed with return demonstration of mixing of proper formula, frequently, and maintenance. Discussed feeding goals, feeding schedule, and techniques.

_____ Instructed on S/S of increased oxygen requirements, and respiratory distress. Interventions discussed such as oxygen via mask and/or nasal cannula.

_____ Instructed with return demonstration oxygen delivery system, how to control flow, read dials, and order oxygen as needed.

Signature/Title of Person Trained: ____________________
Date: ________

Signature/Title of Trainer:__________________________
Date: ________

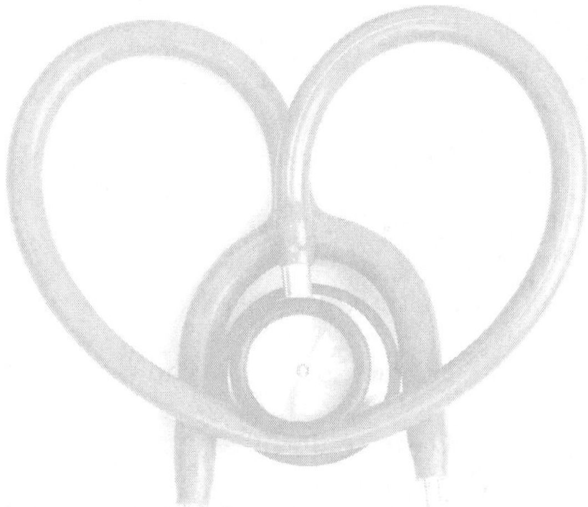

Medical Procedures for Medically Fragile Foster Homes

All the preceding medical interventions were an overview. You will receive individual training for each child prior to taking him or her home. No intervention should be preformed without training by a health care professional. All training needs to be documented.

Administering Enteral Nutrition via Gastrostomy Tube

Infants who are unable to take nourishment by mouth because of conditions such as anomalies of the throat, esophagus, or bowel, impaired swallowing capacity, severe debilitation, respiratory distress, or unconsciousness are frequently fed by way of a tube. This tube is inserted directly into the stomach (gastrostomy) or jejunum (jejunostomy). Such feedings may be intermittent or by continuous drip. Placement of a gastrostomy tube is performed under general anesthesia, and the tube is held in place by a balloon filled with fluid. Care is exercised to prevent excessive pull on the tube that might cause widening of the opening and subsequent leakage of highly irritating gastric juices.

The schedule of tube feedings is planned to meet the infant's nutritional, fluid, and electrolyte needs. A physician must order tube feedings. The order should include formula, rate, route, and frequency. Some tube feedings are ordered as continuous drip over twenty-four hours while others are ordered for a specified amount given at intermittent intervals.

Procedures for Gastrostomy Feedings

Bolus Method

- Elevate head of bed to thirty degrees during the feeding and one hour after to help prevent aspiration.
- You will need a syringe to aspirate stomach contents. This is done when the infant is first

started on feedings. The residual is the contents of the last feeding remaining in the stomach just before the next feeding is to be given. If more than half of the last feeding remains in the stomach as residual, hold feeding for one hour, then check residual again. If the infant continues to have large amounts of residual, hold feedings and contact the doctor.

- Record gastric residual if ordered and return the residual into the stomach.
- Slowly pour the formula into the syringe and unclamp the tubing. Keep the syringe filled to prevent air from entering the stomach. Adjust the flow rate by raising or lowering the syringe. The feeding should finish in five to ten minutes for bolus feedings.
- When the syringe is nearly empty, add the prescribed amount of water to the syringe. Administration of water with gastric feedings also maintains fluid and electrolyte balance.

Continuous drip method

- Hang gavage bag on IV pole.
- Connect administration set to end of gastrostomy tube.
- Connect to infusion pump and set pump.
- Advance tube feedings (as ordered). Should be advanced gradually to prevent diarrhea and gastric intolerance of formula.
- Provide free water as ordered.

Tube feedings provide an excellent environment for bacterial growth, which may lead to gastrointestinal infection. The tubing and the feeding bag should be changed every twenty-four hours. The infant must receive adequate fluid in order for the waste products or protein metabolism to be excreted in the urine. Fluid intake and output must be recorded carefully. The tube should be flushed regularly with water to prevent clogging of the tube.

Gastrointestinal problems are the most common problem associated with tube feedings. Delayed emptying of the stomach is common. Medication that speeds movement in the stomach may be prescribed. Diarrhea is another common complication. The treatment depends on the cause. In many cases, the diarrheas can be treated by changes in the tube feeding, such as diluting the formula or changing the type of formula. Aspiration is a serious complication. Pneumonia can develop if some of the stomach contents enter the lungs. Elevation of the head of the bed to thirty degrees and periodically measuring gastric residual (so that excessive amounts do not accumulate) are ways of preventing aspiration.

Metabolic complications such as fluid and electrolyte imbalance are easily corrected if the infant is carefully monitored. Mechanical problems can result from irritation of the gastrointestinal tract by the tube itself or from clogging of the tube.

A nutrition support team in collaboration with the physician will monitor the infant carefully to see that nutritional goals are being met and to treat complications if they develop. The infant will be weighted regularly.

Fluid and electrolytes are checked, as are other indicators of nutritional status such as serum albumin and transferrin levels, total lymphocyte count, skinfold thickness, and normal rate of growth in children.

Records should be maintained to record amount and type of feeding, the infant's response to tube feeding, patency of tube, and any adverse effects.

Blood Glucose Monitoring

Because of the nature of diabetes and its short- and long-term complications, it's important that you monitor the child's blood sugar. Blood glucose monitoring is an essential part of any diabetes management plan.

Monitoring the child's blood sugar will tell you how his or her body is responding to certain foods, activities, and medications and will help you manage meal and exercise plans. With the data you get from monitoring, you and the doctor can:

- Identify trends in glucose levels
- Identify factors that may cause high or low glucose levels
- Evaluate the impact of food, activity, and medications on the child's diabetes
- Identify where changes in the treatment plan are needed
- Decide what you need to do when the child under your care is sick
- Discuss with child (if possible) whether or not

the feelings they are having are the result of low or high blood glucose or if it is something unrelated to their diabetes

Six steps to proper monitoring:

1. Know the child's blood sugar target.
2. Learn how to check the child's glucose and teach the child if possible.
3. Decide when to check the child's glucose levels and encourage him or her to also express the need.
4. Identify glucose patterns (document).
5. Determine what causes blood glucose changes.
6. Decide what to do to get the child's blood glucose levels back on target.

When to test:

- Ask the doctor or nurse educator how often you should check the blood glucose. Some children need to check several times a day; others may only need to check a few times a week.
- You may want to check at different times of the day to get an idea of how well the treatment program is working.
- Typical times to check are before breakfast, before lunch, before dinner, and before bedtime. Sometimes it is helpful to check blood glucose

one or two hours after a meal to see the effect of food on glucose levels.

There are certain times when you should check blood sugar more often than usual:

- During periods of illness or stress
- When you suspect that the blood glucose is low or high
- When there are changes made in the treatment program, such as a change in medication doses, meal plan or activity
- When the child is taking new medications

Your doctor or diabetes educator will help you choose the glucose meter that is best for you and will teach you and the child how to use it and how to record the results. Several different meters and supplies are available to help you check blood glucose levels.

Important features of a blood glucose meter to consider include:

- Fast results
- Small blood sample size
- Size of meter
- Easy-to-read numbers on display
- Ability to check blood sugar in other places besides finger

- Data management (such as tracking date and time of blood sugar results)
- Cost of supplies and insurance coverage
- How easy is it to use the meter and strips

Checking blood sugar is a simple process using a lancing device, lancet, test strip, and a meter. The diabetes educator will teach you how to do this with the blood glucose meter you have chosen. The following are general instructions for using a blood glucose meter.

- Wash your hands or clean your finger or other site with alcohol. If you are using alcohol, let it dry before you prick the finger.
- Prick the site with a lancing device.
- Put a little drop of blood on a test strip.
- Follow the instructions for inserting the test strip and using the blood glucose meter.
- In seconds, the blood glucose meter reads the blood sugar level.

Supplies you will use:

- Blood glucose meter: reads blood sugar.
- Test strip: collects blood sample.
- Lancet or small needle: fits into lancing device, pricks finger, and provides small drop of blood for glucose strip.

- Lancing device: pricks finger when button is pressed.
- Alcohol wipes or soap and water: clean fingers or other testing site.
- Control solution: checks test strip for accuracy. The amount of sugar in the control solution is already known. When placed on a test strip, the value should match the control solution value on bottle, package of strips, or package insert with your strips.
- User manual: provides information about the meter. After reading it, place the manual in a safe place so that you can find it when you have a question about the meter.
- Warranty card or papers: complete, make a file copy, and send in immediately.

Troubleshooting Tips:

Having problems getting blood out of finger?

- Place hands under warm water and rub together
- Hang hand down below waist
- Grasp finger near area to be pricked and squeeze gently for three seconds
- Place finger on table or firm surface to avoid moving while pricking
- If lancing device has dial-a-depth, increase setting by one level

Child complains that it hurts too much?

- If lancing device has dial-a-depth, decrease setting by one level
- Use new lancet every time you check blood sugar
- Try a thinner lancet or a different lancing device
- Use sides of fingertips instead of fingertip pad
- Try alternative test sites such as arm or thigh
- Ask diabetes educator for suggestions

Error message?

- Review user manual: error codes and problems are identified in manual
- Make sure right amount of blood is on strip
- Make sure blood is on correct part of strip
- Call toll-free manufacturer's number (listed on back of meter and in user manual)
- Ask diabetes educator for suggestions
- Keep a daily record of your blood glucose monitoring in a logbook. Ask your health-care provider for one if you do not already have one.
- Write down the glucose levels in the space provided.
- Write down the medication dose, especially any changes in medication.
- In the note or comment section, write down

changes in food, activity, illness, stress, or insulin reactions.

- Bring the logbook to all appointments with the diabetes health-care providers so they can assess diabetes control.
- Continue to use the logbook even if you're traveling or are on vacation.

In order to get a complete picture of blood glucose levels throughout the day, it is useful to test at different times. The doctor will help you with blood glucose targets. Here is what the numbers can mean. These examples are based upon the American Diabetes Association guidelines.

- Fasting blood glucose before breakfast: This reading on an empty stomach shows how well the child uses the long-acting insulin that he or she takes. The number should be between 90 and 130 mg/dL.
- Premeal blood glucose before lunch and dinner: This reading shows the effectiveness of the breakfast and lunch insulin doses. The number should be between 90 and 130.
- Two hours after eating: The blood glucose peaks a few hours after the child eats. This reading shows if the insulin he or she took was enough to cover the carbs he or she ate. The reading should be less than 180 mg/dL.
- Just before bedtime: A target range for someone with diabetes is 110 to 150 mg/dL. You don't

want to let the child go to bed with blood glucose that is too low because that puts him or her at risk of having a severely low blood sugar episode during the night.

Many doctors ask their patients to report the following information:

- Severely low blood sugar that requires treatment by another person
- Blood sugar consistently running below 70 to 80 more than two to three times in a row
- More than one unexplained low blood sugar reaction in a week
- Blood sugars consistently higher than 300 (more than two to three days)
- If the child is ill with nausea, vomiting, diarrhea or fever

Do not worry if one reading is out of range by a small amount. However, if a number of readings are out of target, then look for a pattern. Does the blood glucose tend to be too high or low at the same time each day? If you spot a pattern, ask the doctor whether you need to adjust food intake, exercise, or medications.

The thought of injecting a child with insulin takes a little getting used to, and doing it properly requires some practice. But once you've made it through the first shot, insulin injection will quickly become a regular part of your daily routine. Injecting at the proper depth is an important part of good injection technique. Most health-care professionals recommend that insulin be injected in the subcutaneous fat, which is the layer of fat just below the skin. If you inject too deep, the insulin could go into muscle, where it's absorbed faster but might not last so long (and it hurts more when you inject into muscle). If the injection isn't deep enough, the insulin goes into the skin, which affects the insulin's onset and duration of action.

Most people pinch up a fold of skin and insert the needle at a ninety-degree angle to the skin fold. To pinch the skin properly, follow these steps:

- Squeeze a couple of inches of skin between your thumb and two fingers, pulling the skin and fat away from the underlying muscle.
- Insert the needle.
- Hold the pinch so the needle doesn't go into the muscle.
- Push the plunger (or button, if you're using a pen) to inject the insulin.
- Release the grip on the skin fold.
- Remove the needle from the skin.

Note that not everyone injects at a ninety-degree angle. If you inject into an area of the body that has less fat, you may need to inject at less than a forty-five-degree angle to avoid injecting into a muscle. The angle you should use to insert the syringe or pen needle into the body depends on body type, the injection site, and the length of the needle that you use. The health-care professional can help you determine the right angle of injection to use.

The body absorbs insulin differently depending on where it is injected. Insulin is absorbed fastest when injected into the subcutaneous tissue in the abdomen (stomach), and somewhat less quickly in the upper arms, thighs, and buttocks/hips. You can use the difference in absorption rates to plan where you're going to inject the insulin. For example, rapid-onset insulin can be injected into the abdomen just before or right after you eat a meal to take advantage of the abdomen's fast absorption rate. NPH insulin can be injected into a different site (arms, thighs, or buttocks) to take advantage of the slower absorption rate while sleeping.

Exercise can also affect the absorption rate. If the child plans to play basketball after injecting, for example, choose a site other than shooting/dribbling arm, since injecting there can increase the absorption rate. If you prefer to inject near a part of the body that will be used when exercising, wait at least forty-five minutes after injecting before starting activity.

Bubbles in the insulin syringe won't harm the child if they're injected into the body, but because they're taking up space in the syringe, they'll prevent him or her from getting the entire insulin dose, and that can make it more difficult to stay in target blood sugar range. There are different ways to avoid bubbles, so ask the health-care provider to recommend one. Here are two suggestions:

- Draw up insulin slowly and steadily. You'll know you're drawing too fast when you see bubbles forming in the syringe. If you do see bubbles, push the insulin back into the bottle and redraw. Do this as many times as needed until the bubbles are gone.
- Draw two more units of insulin into the syringe than you normally need. If you see bubbles, flick the syringe with your thumb and middle finger to make the bubbles rise. You must flick the syringe with some force to get the bubbles to move up, but don't flick too hard, or the needle may bend. Once the bubbles are at the top, or once you have examined the syringe and found no bubbles, push the extra two units of insulin back into the bottle.

If you mix clear and cloudy insulin, you can only remove bubbles from the clear insulin, which is drawn first. You can't remove bubbles after both insulins are in the syringe because when you push insulin back into the bottle of cloudy insulin, you may be pushing clear insulin into the cloudy bottle. This would cause two problems:

- You won't get the full amount of clear insulin that you need.
- It will change the insulin in the cloudy insulin bottle that you will need to inject at a later time (because some clear insulin has been mixed into it).

Catherization of Infant Bladder

The purpose of catherization is the sterile collection of a urine specimen for lab analysis or indwelling for constant drainage of bladder and accurate output measurement.

Special Instructions

- Requires physician's order
- Request assistance from another person
- Restrain infant's legs in froglike position

Equipment

- #6 Foley catheter or #5 or #8 feeding tube
- Sterile catheter kit
- Sterile collection receptacle
- Sterile 5–6 cc syringe with normal saline

Procedure

- Explain procedure to infant in terms he or she can understand if possible.
- Open sterile tray and catheter and check Foley bulb.
- Locate meatus.
- Prep perineum/penis with Betadine.
- Using sterile technique, insert catheter.
- Drain bladder until urine is no longer flowing and dispose of urine if not leaving catheter in place.

- If leaving catheter in place, inflate bulb of catheter using 3 cc NS or air and secure tube with tape.
- Secure catheter to infant leg.
- Attach tubing to suitable drainage system.
- Record procedure and indicate results. Chart infant's tolerance.
- Observe meticulous sterile technique to prevent introduction of bacteria into the bladder.
- Clean technique is used if catherization is done regularly.
- Use correct size catheter to prevent bladder spasm and trauma to urethra.

Chest Therapy (CPT)

CPT is used to loosen mucus in the lungs so the baby can cough it up. Certain body positions and percussion (clapping) are used to loosen mucus and help expand collapsed areas of the baby's lung.

Lungs are two balloonlike organs located in chest. The right lung has three lobes. The left lung has two lobes.

Clapping and Vibration

- Clapping is done holding the hand in a cupped manner with all the fingertips and thumbs together.
- In a small baby, clapping may be done holding two or three fingers together and tapping the chest or by using an infant percussor.

- Clapping is done firmly at a fairly fast rate.
- Baby should have blanket or shirt over skin.
- Clapping loosens mucus from lungs. It stimulates the baby to cough and bring up secretions.
- Vibration is done after clapping to stimulate the flow of secretions.
- To vibrate, the hand is kept flat and pressed firmly against same area of chest. The result is described as a controlled quiver. Fingers placed flat against chest wall of small baby may be enough to produce the same effect.
- About one to two minutes should be spent over one area.
- Vibration with padded electric toothbrush or small hand vibrator may be used.
- Coughing may occur shortly afterward. Suction the baby with a bulb syringe.
- The treatment should last no longer than ten minutes.
- Position baby in your lap or on bed using pillows for support.

When To Do CPT

- As ordered by doctor
- Primarily early morning and prior to bedtime
- Before meals or one to one and a half hours after feeding to prevent vomiting

- Caregivers should contact physician if baby requires CPT more often than ordered
- Many babies enjoy CPT. They often fall asleep or become quiet during therapy.

Signs of Tiring or Distress

- Baby becomes blue or pale.
- Baby becomes floppy or limp.
- Baby's breathing becomes difficult or increases in rate.

Problems

- Breathing difficulties
- Aspiration (breathes mucus or formula into the lungs)
- Vomiting
- A pause in the baby's breathing from a blocked airway
- Bruising
- Broken ribs
- Decreased oxygen.
- Injury and/or bleeding of liver or spleen

Be careful! Be gentle!

- Use only battery-operated, electrically safe vibrators.

- Do not apply vibration or percussion to broken skin.
- Avoid positions that will cause breathing problems. Examples of this are:
    - Placing the baby flat or with his head down when his stomach is full
    - Sitting baby up without head support and with his neck bent forward, blocking his breathing passage
- Avoid clapping over fractures, stomach, backbone, or recent chest surgery areas

After CPT, the baby may cough up mucus. Suction his mouth and nose using a bulb syringe. The doctor will determine how long the baby needs CPT.

Colostomy Procedure

The purpose is to prevent leakage of fecal material.

Postoperatively, there is no fecal drainage until approximately two or three days post-op, and the infant/child generally comes from surgery with dry dressing.

Equipment

- Approximate appliance, karaya seal, and stoma bag. Bags come in different sizes from three-quarter inch to three inches
- Stoma measuring card
- Washcloth and mild soap

- Stomahesive, if needed
- Ostomy belt, if desired
- Gloves

Procedure

- Put on gloves.
- Obtain accurate bag by measuring stoma with card.
- Examine stoma for discoloration, edema, lacerations, or prolapse.
- Thoroughly clean the area around the stoma by washing with lukewarm soapy water, rinsing well, and patting it dry. This will help prevent skin irritation around the stoma.
- Apply stomahesive if excessive drainage is causing frequent bag changes or poor adhesive of appliance. This is used to protect the skin against drainage by providing an effective skintight adhesive. Remains intact for up to seven days.
- Cut stomahesive to fit snugly around stoma without causing pressure. Press firmly into the skin.
- Apply correct size karaya seal bag. Bag can be changed once a day, unless there is excessive fecal drainage, which requires more frequent bag changes.
- Peel protective covering and press karaya bag firmly against skin with stomahesive.

- Fold bottom of bag to collect drainage and apply clamp.
- Attach ostomy belt to secure the bag, especially during ambulation.
- Remove gloves and wash hands.
- Document ostomy care and pertinent observations in progress notes.

Enemas for Infants and Children

The purpose of enemas is to promote emptying of the colon and/or instill medication.

Equipment

- Infant enema set (syringe and rectal tube) for children under one year
- Regular enema set for children over one year.
- Lubricant
- Adequate linen or underpads to protect the bed and prevent unnecessary exposure of child
- Graduated container for measuring fluid

Special Information

- The doctor orders the type and amount of solution to be used.
- If the doctor does not specify the amount of solution to be used, the following may be used as a guide:

- Newborn to six months: 50–100 cc
- Six to eighteen months: 100–150 cc
- Nineteen to twenty-four months: 150–200 cc
- Two to three years: 200–300 cc
- Three to four years: 300–400 cc
- Four to six years: 400–500 cc
- Six to twelve years: 500–750 cc
- Twelve years and over: 750–1000 cc

Solutions

- Normal saline: use saline for irrigation
- Soap suds: 1cc castile soap to each 100 cc of water
- Commercial enema: use pediatric size
- Retention enema: mineral oil or medication as ordered

Procedure

- Explain the procedure to infant or child in terms the child can understand if possible. Provide privacy.
- Enlist assistance of another person as necessary.
- Place underpads under buttocks.
- Position child on left side with knees flexed on abdomen.

- Lubricate tip of rectal tube, expel air from tubing, and gently insert the tube into the rectum.
- Raise the solution eight to ten inches above the level of the child's hips and let the solution run by gravity.
- If the child is able to cooperate, the noncommercial cleansing enemas should be retained three to five minutes.
- Place the child on the bedpan, potty-chair, or toilet. Diaper the infant securely.

Documentation

- Medication record
- VS/I&O sheet.
- Record in child's notes

All children will be considered contagious, and preventive measures will be carried out to prevent unnecessary exposure to blood and body fluids.

Gastrostomy Tube

A gastrostomy tube (GT) is a way to feed babies who are not able to suck or swallow enough for good nutrition. The gastrostomy tube is placed directly into the stomach. Babies who have a GT may have a problem with his or her heart, esophagus, mouth (such as a cleft palate), may be on a ventilator for a long time, or may not be able to suck and/or swallow well.

The button gastrostomy has a one-way valve inside that makes it difficult for milk to come out of the stomach and button. Babies who have problems with gas may not do well with this type of gastrostomy. A special tube fits in the button to feed the baby. The tube is removed and the outside flap closed after each feeding.

Advantages of the Button

You remove the feeding tube after the feeding.

- It looks better.
- Tube care is easy. You do not need to measure the tube or use special adhesive dressings.
- There are fewer skin problems.
- It lasts longer. Generally, it lasts three to four months before it needs to be replaced. The one-way valve not working is the most common reason the button needs to be changed.

Disadvantages of the Button

- You must take the baby to the doctor if the button comes out if you are not willing to learn to replace it yourself. A Foley catheter is placed in the stoma until another button can be inserted. You will receive a Foley catheter from the physician when the button is surgically placed. Learning to replace the button yourself is very simple after the stoma is healed.
- The valve that stops formula from coming up feeding tube may get clogged and stop working.

- The feeding tube can come disconnected if baby is active during feeding

Inserting the Button

- The button may be inserted in the surgery doctor's office or in the hospital.
- Your baby is given pain medicine before the button is inserted. It stings when the stoma is stretched before the button is placed.
- The doctor uses a guide to stretch the button out so it can be inserted through the stoma and into the stomach.
- Your baby will be fussy several hours after the button is inserted. The doctor may have you use Tylenol or pain medicine to make the baby comfortable. He will recover by the next day.
- The stoma may be weepy or bleed slightly the first day or two.
- Turn the button in a complete circle each time you feed the baby the first three to four days after the button is placed.

Skin care: Cleaning the stoma (opening)

Supplies

- Mild soap cloth to wash skin
- Water cloth to dry skin
    - Wash the skin with mild soap and water one to two times a day.

- Dry the skin well and leave open to air for about fifteen minutes.
- Turn the button in a complete circle one to two times a day.

Weepy Skin (Method 1)

- If the skin is weepy or blistered, rinse the area well with water and pat dry.
- Sprinkle Stomahesive powder on weepy skin. (The doctor will order it.)
- Dust off extra powder. Stomahesive powder will stick to weepy skin.
- Repeat every three to four days until skin is healed.
- Call the doctor if the area is not better in one week.

Weepy Skin (Method 2)

- If the skin is weepy or blistered, rinse the area well with water and pat dry.
- Apply a thin layer of barrier cream.
- Call the doctor if the area is not better in one week.

Rash: If skin looks like it has prickly heat or diaper rash, wash the area with soap and water. Rinse well and pat dry.

- Apply a thin coat of Aseptin or Micro-Guard cream (doctor will order).
- Massage the cream into the skin and let dry.
- Repeat every two to three days until skin is healed.
- Call the doctor if the area is not better in one week.

Button Care

- Flush the tube and button with 2 to 5 cc of tap water after each feeding. This will stop the button from getting clogged up as easily.
- Clean the inside of the button with a Q-Tip and tap water daily.

Types of Feeding Tubes

- Decompression tube: Longer end to vent and decompress stomach (opening on the side). Should not be used for feedings.
- Feeding tube for continuous: End is shorter. Use for regular or continuous feedings. Smaller size tubing allows for more control. Does not open one-way valve, so no venting occurs.
- Feeding tube for bolus: Tubing is larger. Opening is at the end of the tube. Used for thicker fluids. Difficult to control the rate of the feeding. Does not open the one-way valve, so no venting occurs.

Feeding Supplies

- Gather all equipment before beginning feeding:
- Formula in 60 cc catheter tip syringe
- Pacifier
- Tap water
- Make baby comfortable: change diaper, suction if needed, offer pacifier, place in infant seat or on bed with head elevated.
- Attach feeding tube adapter to button.
- Check for formula left in stomach from last feeding (residuals) by attaching a syringe to the tube and gently pulling back on plunger. Give this material back to your baby. Do not throw this away. It contains important nutrients. If more than 15 to 20 cc of formula are present, call the doctor for a possible change in feedings.
- Remove the plunger from the syringe. Put the syringe into the open end of the feeding tube.
- Pinch feeding tube closed. Hold syringe upright.
- Pour formula into the syringe and add any medications. Release the tube and let the feeding begin to flow. Some parents measure formula for each feeding into a plastic bottle instead of directly into syringe.
- Add more formula as the syringe empties. Pinch the tube closed when adding more formula. To

prevent air from getting into the stomach, do not let syringe run dry.

- Feeding should run at 2 to 3 cc per minute or be finished in about twenty minutes.
- To start the feeding, a gentle push with the plunger may be needed.
- Feeding should flow by gravity slowly (hold syringe above the baby)!
- When feeding is finished, flush with 5 cc of tap water or air to clear it of formula.
- Remove feeding tube and close flap. Formula should not come back up the button because it has a one-way valve.
- Baby may need to be burped.
- After feeding, place baby on right side with his or her body propped at a thirty-degree angle.
- Clean equipment by washing syringe and feeding tube with hot soapy water. Let it air dry. Store in clean towel or baggie.
- Tube feedings are not to be hung or left unattended.
- If feeding tube comes off button, formula will pour out on the baby. Put tube back on and re-feed amount of formula you think was lost.

Medications

- Thick medicines can clog the button. They need to be diluted with water or formula before being placed in the syringe.

- Medicine in tablet form must be crushed and mixed with water or formula before being placed in the syringe.
- Give medicines in beginning of the feeding. The remainder of the feeding can wash all the medicine down the tube.
- Flush feeding tube and button with 2 to 5 cc of tap water at the end of feeding.

Cleaning and storing equipment

- Wash the feeding tube in hot soapy water, rinse well, and air dry after each feeding.
- Store in clean towel or baggie.

Mouth Care:

It may be necessary to clean the baby's nose and mouth with finger cloth and warm water.

Call the doctor if:

- Bloody residuals (formula left in baby's stomach between feedings)
- Residuals greater than 15–20 ccs
- Stomach enlargement not helped by attaching feeding tube and hanging the tube open for one hour
- Leaking formula
- Tissue buildup around the gastrostomy tube
- Unpleasant smell from the stoma (opening

into stomach), bleeding stoma, formula leaking around gastrostomy tube

- Button is clogged and formula will not go down tube. Attempt to flush 5 cc of tap water down tube. Use very gentle pressure on plunger. Stop if formula does not flow easily.

Other Information

- You may hold the baby during the feeding when you feel more comfortable with feeding your baby by gastrostomy.
- Feeding by nipple should be tried before gastrostomy feeding when the baby is allowed to nipple part or all of his feeding.
- If the baby does not feed by bottle or takes most of his feedings by tube, you may give the one or two night feedings by gastrostomy tube, particularly if the baby is asleep or not alert. As the baby's nipple feedings increase, these feedings can be fed by bottle.

Increasing Feedings

- The doctor will give you a schedule on how to increase the baby's feedings. Feedings are increased according to weight gained and calories needed for growth.
- Feedings are usually increased about 5 cc for each half pound of weight gained.

- Baby should be weighed once a week either at the doctor's office or you can use your own baby scale.
- You should use a feeding record (see sample forms) to keep track of how well the baby eats. Take this record with you to each doctor's visit.

Supplies:

- All of the home supplies you need for the first month will be sent home with you. The hospital makes these arrangements with a company near where you live.
- The supply company will contact you at home or as arranged.
- The supply company will tell you when to re-order supplies, or you can call them to reorder supplies.
- Medical is the insurance that most foster children are covered with. The supply company will inform you about the supplies that are covered. If the child needs something that is not covered and the doctor orders it, contact the baby's social worker, and he or she will attempt to cover the extra costs. He or she can work with the supply company to make sure you have what the baby needs.
- You need to order new tubes about every six months or if the adapter that goes into the button does not fit well. You are sent home with extra tubes.

If the gastrostomy tube falls out, do not panic. If the stoma is new (the tube has been in for less than six weeks):

- Cover the stoma with a clean gauze or cloth.
- You need to have a doctor put the tube back in as soon as possible (within two hours).
- The stoma will close pretty quickly (we usually say four to six hours).
- Oftentimes, an X-ray with contrast (dye) will be taken to make sure the tube is in the right place before feeds can be restarted.

If the stoma is more than six weeks old:

- You need to place a feeding tube into the stoma as soon as possible.
- PEGs and Bard buttons cannot be replaced. You will have to use the Foley catheter from your emergency kit.
- Mic-Key (button) can be reinserted.
- Always make sure you get stomach contents returned before restarting feeds.

Remember to always carry a replacement tube with you. You will need to place the tube into the stoma to stop the tract/hole from closing.

Steps to Reinserting the Gastrostomy Tube

Gather equipment:

- Feeding tube (Foley catheter or skin level tube)
- Washcloth
- Tape
- 5 ml syringe to inflate the balloon
- 5 ml water to inflate the balloon
- Water soluble lubricant (like KY Jelly)

How to reinsert tube

- Draw up 5 ml of water into the syringe.
- Check the balloon on the new tube before putting it into the stoma by inflating the balloon with 5 ml of water.
- Deflate the balloon by pulling the water back into the syringe.
- Moisten the end of the tube with water or water-soluble lubricant (to make the tube go in easier).
- Insert the new tube about two inches into the stoma.
- Inflate balloon with the 5 ml of water in the syringe, then remove the empty syringe from the tube.
- Gently pull back on the tube to feel it snug against the stomach wall.

- Clean and dry the skin and tape the tube to the skin to secure.
- If using a catheter, you should mark where the tube comes out of the body; you can use this as a checkmark for placement.
- Check the placement of the tube by withdrawing stomach contents and make sure this fluid goes back into the stomach.
- If unable to withdraw stomach contents, reposition and try again. If you cannot get any stomach contents then wait half an hour and try again. If you're unsure that the tube is in the stomach, do not use the tube.

Guidelines for Infant/Child with Fever and Temperature Taking

Fever, one of the most common symptoms of illness in children, is also one of the most frequent misunderstood manifestations of disease and a great source of concern to parents and caretakers. If fever persists or reaches an unacceptable level defined by the physician, implement sponging with tepid water and administer antipyretics as ordered. Fever is an adaptive response of the body and seems to form host defense. Recent studies show fever has beneficial effects, including inhibition of bacterial growth and enhanced motility of white blood cells. The physician will often prescribe an acceptable temperature range.

The child is observed for:

- Rapid heartbeat
- A full, bounding pulse or a weak, thready pulse
- Rapid breathing
- Hot, dry skin
- Chills or sweating
- Headache
- Dehydration
- Tremors

Treatment may include, per MD order, giving antibiotic, antifever, and sedative drugs. If the temperature is extremely high, a cooling tub bath, a cool wet sheet, or small ice packs may be helpful. The child's temperature is checked every two to four hours. Increased amounts of fluids are given, physical activity is reduced, and the skin is exposed to air. Remove excess cloths, blankets, or bed coverings. Environmental measures to reduce fever are used if tolerated by the child and if they do not induce shivering.

Shivering is the body's way of maintaining the set point by producing heat. Controlling the environment, such as minimal clothing, exposing the skin to the air, reducing room temperature and increasing air circulation can be very effective. In addition, cool moist compresses to the skin, such as the forehead, are most effective if employed approximately one hour after an antipyretic (such as Tylenol) is given so that the hypothalamic set point is lowered.

There are three ways to take a temperature:

- Auxiliary (armpit): takes three to four minutes to register. This method may be used in babies under six months or children up to four years.
- Rectal (in the bottom): takes two to three minutes to register. This method may be used in children over six months and less than six years.
- Oral (mouth): takes two to three minutes to register. Child should be cooperative and over four years old to use this method.

Thermometers

- There are two types of thermometers: oral and rectal.
- The oral thermometer's bulb is long and thin.
- The rectal thermometer's bulb is round so it will not be sharp against the walls of the rectum.
- The markings on both thermometers are identical.

Taking a Temperature

- Take the temperature when your baby is quiet, if possible.
- Body temperature varies depending on the amount of activity, emotional stress, and type of clothing worn, and temperature of the environment.
- When reporting fever, always tell the doctor the exact thermometer reading and where the temperature was taken.

- We recommend using the auxiliary (armpit) temperature on babies less than six months of age.
- If using a digital thermometer, press power button and wait until display appears. This indicates the unit is operational and in good condition. Follow the directions for taking a temperature.
- If you are using a glass thermometer, make sure the thermometer has been shaken down before taking the baby's temperature. If the mercury (shiny band) is above 96 degrees Fahrenheit, shake it down by holding the thermometer and snapping the wrist sharply.
- Check to make sure the bulb of the thermometer is not broken or cracked.

Generally, fever is a temperature over 99 degrees Fahrenheit if taken in the armpit or over 100 degrees Fahrenheit if taken rectally. Ask your doctor when he or she would like to be notified if the child has a fever.

Reading a Thermometer

- Find the silver line in the thermometer.
- Hold the thermometer at eye level.
- Turn it slowly until you see the scale markings on top and the numbers on the bottom.
- You will see a shiny band between the markings on the top and the numbers on the bottom.
- Be sure not to hold the end with the bulb when reading the thermometer!

- Read the number at the end of the shiny band. This is the temperature reading.

Taking an Auxiliary Temperature (under arm)

- Use any thermometer.
- Hold the thermometer snugly in the armpit, making sure the bulb is completely covered between your baby's arm and side.
- Hold the thermometer there for three to four minutes.
- Remove from under the arm and read the thermometer (shiny band) or digital window.
- When reporting your baby's temperature, tell the nurse or doctor that it was an auxiliary temperature.
- Auxiliary temperatures are slightly lower than rectal or oral temperatures.

Taking a Rectal Temperature (in the bottom):

- Select a thermometer with a stubby-type bulb.
- Shake mercury down past 96 degrees Fahrenheit.
- Moisten lower portion of thermometer with Vaseline or KY Jelly.
- Place infant on his stomach and across your lap.
- Spread the buttocks with one hand to expose the anal opening and lay that arm along your baby's back to prevent him from moving.

- Insert thermometer with your other hand, slowly and gently, just far enough for bulb to pass the anal sphincter (muscle). This is about one inch.
- Hold thermometer in place for approximately two to three minutes.
- Remove gently in a straight line and read it.

Care of Thermometer

- Draw thermometer through soapy cotton ball or tissue.
- Rinse in cool water.
- Store in safe place, out of the reach of children.

Call the doctor if:

- Baby has fever over 100 degrees Fahrenheit auxiliary (under arm) or 101 degrees Fahrenheit rectal, and/or vague symptoms:
    - Irritability (crying or fussy)
    - Poor feeding
    - Floppy or listless (call 911)
    - Breathing is difficult (call 911)
    - Coughing
    - Does not look good.
- Temperature is less than 97 degrees Fahrenheit.
- If your baby feels hot to touch and you are unable to read a thermometer.

- Fever is present for more than three days or as ordered.
- Fever with abnormal movements.

Remember, a normal temperature is around 98 degrees Fahrenheit.

Treating Fever

- If your baby is less than six months of age and has a fever, call the baby's doctor before giving acetaminophen (Tylenol, Tempera, Liquiprin, Panadol, or Ibuprofen/Advil, with MD order only)
- Get the correct dosage from your baby's doctor.
- Do not use medicine for more than three days without talking with the doctor.
- Keep all medicine out of the reach of children.
- Children should not be given aspirin. Several studies link aspirin use in children with Reye's syndrome, a severe illness that often is fatal.

Hand Washing

Hand washing is the single most important preventive measure against infection. The caretaker must perform thorough hand washing before and after all contact with the infant, as well as before and after performing specific procedures. The Center for Disease Control recommends that individuals in contact with infants who require special care should routinely wash their hands in the following situations:

- Before and after contact with an infant (particularly those with high susceptibility to infection)
- After touching organic material (like changing a diaper)
- Before and after performing invasive procedures such as injections or tracheal suctioning
- Before and after handling dressings or touching open wounds
- Before and after handling contaminated equipment
- Before and after preparing medications
- May need gloves for infectious items or illness such as HIV positive

Before a caretaker begins working with infant, hand washing for one minute provides good protection. A thirty-second hand washing after each routine contact helps to minimize microorganism spread. Hand washing is required before caretaker works with sterile equipment. A one-minute hand washing is also recommended whenever caretaker has handled contaminated equipment or organic material.

Ostomy Skin Care

Ostomy is a general term for an operation in which an artificial opening is formed, as in colostomy, ureterostomy, gastrostomy, and tracheotomy. Because the skin is the infant's first line of defense against infection, skin-care practices are of special importance. After healing takes place, meticulous care is needed to keep the area surrounding the tube (the stoma) clean and dry to prevent excoriation and infection.

- Always wash your hands with warm, soapy water before touching the ostomy tube.
- Develop a habit of inspecting the skin around the tube (stoma) after feeding, suctioning, or changing the ostomy bag.
- Make sure the skin is clean and dry. Observe the stoma for a few minutes, checking for gastric leakage or air leak (trach).
- If you use a dressing, change it when it becomes wet or soiled. Never allow a wet dressing to remain in contact with the skin. (Most G-tubes or trachs do not require a dressing after site is healed.)
- Gently clean the skin around the tube. Use cotton-tipped applicators or a soft cloth with soap and warm water. Rotate the G-tube and clean again.
- Remove dry, crusted secretions with gauze or cotton-tipped applicators saturated with half-strength hydrogen peroxide. If you think soap is irritating the skin, try cleansing with water alone, or try another soap.
- Powders and lotions must not be used around tube opening. An ointment can be applied in a thin layer to treat irritations or rashes.

The human body tends to heal; therefore, treatment of rashes or irritations is best directed toward eliminating influences that interfere with normal healing processes. The most common offenders in infants are environmental factors such as soaps, bubble baths, shampoos, rough or tight clothing, blankets, toys, and the natural elements such as dirt, sand, heat, cold, moisture, and wind.

Tracheostomy Care and Suctioning

Since the normal warming, wetting, and filtering junctions of the upper airway are inoperative, air entering the tracheostomy opening is humidified by attaching a special mask or collar to deliver humidified air directly to the trach opening. The humid air helps to loosen mucus and reduce the chances of crust formation and a mucous plug. Moisture from the humidified air tends to accumulate on the inner surface of the flexible plastic tubing and must be eliminated periodically to prevent occlusion of the tube and/or accidental aspiration. An infant may need to have mist treatments at least three to four times a day and all during the night. If the baby has difficulty with suctioning or mucus plugs, more mist treatments may be required.

When to suction trach:

- Loud gurgles are heard in trach tube
- Bubbles are noticed in the trach
- Rattles are felt on the baby's back or chest
- Baby seems agitated, restless, cries, and cannot be quieted
- Increased breathing rate or increased heart rate
- Baby becomes pale or blue

- Flaring nostrils (move in and out when breathing)
- Suction only as needed

After inserting one or two normal saline drops, suction by blocking the fingerhole and withdrawing the catheter slowly. Rotate the catheter between your fingers to get better suctioning of the trach. Do not cover suction catheter fingerhole when inserting the suction catheter. Suctioning should last only three to five seconds during each entry. Suctioning may have to be repeated after inserting more normal saline. If possible, try not to suction for at least thirty minutes after meals. Change suction catheter at the beginning of each eight hours. Use clean technique during suctioning. Rinse out suction container at the end of each eight hours.

Counting Baby's Breathing

- You may want to count the baby's breathing rate twice a day when the baby is quiet or asleep. You can write the number in a record book you bring to the doctor.
- One count is a breath in and out. Sometimes the baby holds his breath briefly, breathes fast then slow, stretches or moves. Count the breathing as best you can.
- Call the doctor if the breathing rate is fifteen to twenty counts higher than usual or your baby is working harder to breathe. Make sure the baby is not too warm or does not have mucus in his trach.

Cleaning the Tracheostomy Opening (Stoma): The area around the tracheostomy opening in the neck is cleaned daily, trach ties are changed as needed, and the trach tube is changed as per MD order.

- Support the trach tube with a finger while cleaning.
- Wet Q-tip in half-strength hydrogen peroxide and roll Q-tip over skin, under trach tube, and move outward to remove crusted secretions.
- Rinse with Q-tip dipped in clean water.
- Pat dry with clean cloth.
- Wash skin around neck with a mild soap daily.
- Change trach dressing as often as necessary to keep skin dry and clean.
- Clean stoma BID (twice a day) or more often if an odor is present. Powders and lotions must not be used around trach opening. An ointment can be applied in a thin layer to treat irritations or rashes.

Inserting New or Cleaned Trach

- If possible, never change a trach tube alone. It is always safer to have two persons change a trach tube together.
- Always suction before changing trach and immediately afterwards.
- Place a small towel behind infant's neck to help lift chin and make changing the trach easier.
- Untie trach strings of the old trach and place

small amount of surgical lubricant on end of new trach.

- Remove old trach with one hand using an up-and-out motion (follow angle of tube).
- Insert new or cleaned tube gently. Direct tube back and down.
- Remove obturator as soon as the tube is in place; then secure ties. The infant cannot breathe unless the guide (obturator) is removed.
- Clean trach tube as instructed and place into small baggie for future use.

An infant with a tracheostomy requires continuous attendance. An infant or small child must be placed under direct observation at all times or must be placed on a cardiac/apnea monitor continuously while not under direct observation. Any problem or sign or symptom of infection must be reported to the RN or physician.

Attention must be given to ensure that infants with a tracheostomy are well hydrated to keep secretions loose enough for removal by cough or suction. In addition, these infants frequently use more calories than normal; therefore they need to have nutritionally sound diets and may require high-calorie supplements. The infant's weight and height will be measured (recorded) regularly. Because they have more difficulty generating sufficient pressure on expiration to remove secretions effectively, chest physiotherapy and postural drainage may be a regular part of care to help mobilize secretions. These measures are used anytime suctioning is unable to clear deeper-situated secretions.

Emergency Procedures

If the baby stops breathing:

- Suction trach tube at once.
- Replace trach tube if it has come out, is blocked with mucus, and/or baby does not improve with suctioning.
- Begin CPR if baby does not breathe when trach tube is clear by placing mouth or attaching ambu bag over trach tube to form seal.
- Give two quick puffs. Observe to see if chest moves like an easy breath.
- Continue with CPR if needed and call 911.

"Go bag" for traveling:

- Suction catheter
- Bulb syringe
- Suction catheters that are disposable
- Trach tube with tie and obturator (same size and size smaller)
- Scissors
- Water-soluble lubricant (sterile single-use packets)
- Saline (two to three 5 cc vials)
- 4 x 4s or trach sponges

- Portable suction machine
- Emergency phone numbers

Safety Tips

- Keep home as free from lint and dust as possible.
- Do not use powders, chlorine bleach, ammonia, or aerosol sprays in the same room as the baby. Particles and fumes get into the lungs through the trach. This will cause a burning feeling and breathing problems.
- Do not smoke around the baby. Smoke is irritating to the baby's windpipe (trachea).
- Watch play with other children so that toys, fingers, and food are not put into trach tube.
- Always carry your "go bag" supplies when you leave home.

Weather

- During freezing temperature, avoid allowing baby to breathe cold air directly into trach. This can cause a tracheal spasm and form small ice particles in the mucus if exposed for long periods of time. Keep the baby's head and neck loosely covered with a blanket. Tie a scarf loosely around the neck of an older child.
- Protect the tracheostomy on dusty windy days when dust particles may enter the trachea and cause drying or crusting mucus.

Making Sounds and Talking

- At first you will not be able to hear the baby cry or make sounds. This is because the air from the lungs does not pass through the vocal cords.
- He will learn to talk around the trach tube.
- It is important that you talk to him as you would any other baby.

More Information

- The baby may have trach collar and humidity off during the day if allowed by the baby's doctor.
- Use trach collar and humidity during naps and at night to keep trach moist and prevent mucus plugs.
- If a humidifier is not available (during long trips or power failure), place one drop of saline every hour or two into the trach tube to moisten trach tube and windpipe.
- The windpipe (trachea) of the baby is small and easily plugged with mucus, so the humidifier with trach collar provides a direct source of moisture that a vaporizer cannot.
- If mucus becomes thick, move the numbered ring on the humidifier to a lower number. The usual setting is 50 percent. Increasing the baby's fluid intake may help thin the mucus.
- A humidifier and tracheostomy collar (trach collar) are used to filter and moisten air entering

the windpipe (trachea) because the baby does not breathe through his nose or mouth.

Cleaning Procedure for Tracheotomy Tubes

- Place the used tracheotomy tube and obturator in a bowl.
- Pour hydrogen peroxide into the bowl until all pieces are completely covered.
- Using the nonabrasive brush or pipe cleaners, gently cleanse and remove any secretions that may be on the outside or inside of the tube and obturator.
- Hold tube over sink or bowel and rinse with sterile water, being sure to thoroughly rinse off any hydrogen peroxide. Do the same for the obturator.
- Air dry the tracheostomy tubes and obturator on a paper towel. With the parts completely dry, place a plastic bag, seal closed, and store ready for your next tracheostomy tube change.
- Clean the trach ties with soap and water and let air dry on the counter; then store with clean trach for the next use. Do not place into the washer. It will ruin the ties.

Clean Storage of Suction Catheters

- When you have finished suctioning the baby, rinse the catheter by suctioning water through the catheter; then carefully disconnect the catheter and place it in the inside of your glove and store in holder on the side of the bed. The catheter can be stored in this way until the baby requires suctioning again.

- When the baby needs to be suctioned, reconnect the catheter to the connective tubing, being careful not to touch the tip of the catheter.
- Before inserting the catheter into the baby's tracheostomy tube, rinse it once in the water (suction cup). The catheter can now be used to suction the baby's tracheostomy tube.

A new suction catheter should be used every eight hours or more frequently for a baby with increased amounts of secretions. The suction cup needs to be cleaned or changed every time a new, clean catheter is used.

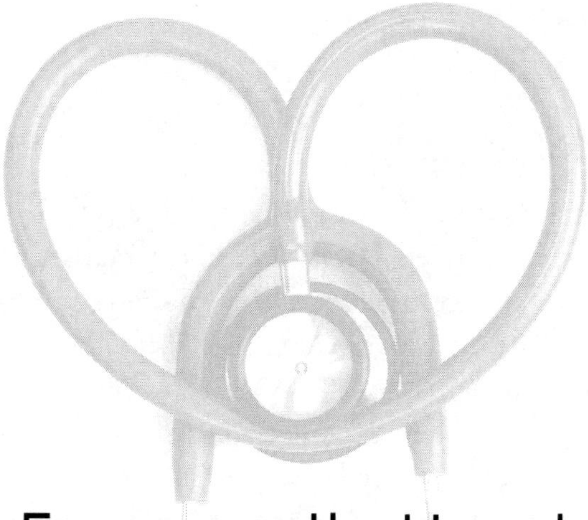

Frequently Used Medical Equipment for the Medically Fragile Child

Air Compressor

Air compressors are used to turn liquid into a mist so that it can be inhaled. It is used for patients who have a tracheostomy or otherwise need to deliver a mist that moisturizes their airway. The mist keeps the secretions from becoming too thick. When breathing through a tracheostomy, the air no longer passes through the nose where it normally would be warmed, filtered, and humidified. Because of this, most trach patients require an air compressor that humidifies the air delivered to the trach and lungs. Occasionally heaters are added to increase the humidity output and to warm the air. Although air compressor equipment may vary in appearance, most models operate in a similar fashion.

Most patients will use the air compressor when they are in bed at night or during naps. Always make sure that the air compressor is kept below the level of the patient's head to prevent aspiration of any accumulated water in the tubing.

How to use:

- Fill the humidifier jar with distilled water.
- Attach the humidifier jar to output arm of the air compressor.
- Attach a length of corrugated aerosol tubing to the humidifier jar.
- Attach a water drainage bag or washable water trap to the end of the aerosol tubing.

- Attach a second length of aerosol tubing onto the other side of the drainage bag.
- Attach a trach mask to the end of the aerosol tubing.
- Turn the on switch on the air compressor and set the pressure dial on the front between 23 and 25 psi, or as instructed by the respiratory therapist.
- You should see a fine mist coming through the tubing and out through the trach mask. The amount of mist produced by the compressor can be adjusted by rotating the dial.

This is an overview on an air compressor. For complete instructions, be sure to read the patient instructions that will be provided with the air compressor. Also, see the manual for oxygen delivery, heated humidity, and/or medications delivery via air compressor.

Care and cleaning of the air compressor

- Rinse the jar used for trach mist daily.
- Wash the jar in a nonlotion dishwashing detergent twice weekly.
- Rinse the sponge filter in clean water. Dry thoroughly before putting the filter back on the air compressor weekly.

Apnea Monitors

An apnea monitor counts the baby's breathing and heart rate. It is used to alert the care provider if either is out of the normal range.

Cautions

- Ensure you know and are comfortable performing CPR.
- Identify another person (family member or neighbor) to be able to provide assistance if you need it to call 911, etc.
- Post your address, major cross streets, and medications by the telephone so the information is available to the person making the emergency call.
- Use monitor whenever the care provider is asleep or whenever the baby is in another room or whenever the baby is sleeping.
- Observe skin under the leads or belt for signs of redness or irritation. If observed, move leads or belt to another location on the chest. Notify doctor if irritation continues.
- Keep a monitor alarm log; it will help doctor decide if/when the baby needs a medication and/or when it is safe to discontinue its use.
- Do not discontinue use without a doctor's order.

Alarms

- The doctor will prescribe the alarm settings, which will be set by the equipment supplier.
- Normal alarm settings (the monitor will alarm if rates are outside these limits):
    - Apnea alarm set at twenty seconds
    - Low heart rate alarm at eighty beats per minute
    - High heart rate alarm at 250 beats per minute

Other alarms

- Loose lead, most often cause of alarm
- Belt or wires off or too loose

If machine alarms: Always look at the baby first!

- If the baby is not breathing, proceed with CPR.
- If the baby is breathing and alarm is still sounding, check for loose or disconnected leads or if battery charge is low.
- If the monitor is alarming and there are no loose or disconnected leads, be sure skin beneath leads is clean and does not have lotion on it. A drop or two of water on the lead (on the side that touches baby's skin) may be needed to help make good contact. Also, check the belt placement; if the belt has moved, alarm may sound.

- If you continue to hear alarms and the baby appears okay, contact the equipment company for assistance.
- Follow the manual for further instructions.

Oxygen

Early planning and careful preparation are the keys to bringing home a child with oxygen. Ask the doctor for complete written instructions on:

- How often (e.g. only when asleep, continuous, only when feeding, etc.)
- Liter flow (one-fourth liter per minute, half minute). If a child needs more than two liters per minute, he or she should be in a hospital, so do not accept a child with that high a flow rate.
- If the prescribed flow rate of oxygen is less than one liter per minute, a special pediatric regulator is used. The pediatric regulator has settings for very low flows, such as 1/16, 1/8, and 1/4.
- If a humidifier is required (you should always use a humidifier except for short periods, such as going for a doctor appointment; do not use humidifier with the portable tank or E-bottle).
- Oxygen equipment (find out the source of the oxygen-concentrator—electrical plug in unit size of small refrigerator, or H-bottle size).

It is very important to get hands-on training from a respiratory therapist before bringing the child home.

Cautions

- Oxygen will not burst into flames, but will aid in igniting combustible materials.
- Keep oxygen at least ten feet from heaters, radiators, and appliances with pilot lights.
- No smoking, striking matches, cigarette lighters in vicinity of oxygen.
- Keep hands free of any oil, grease, or petroleum products, such as Vaseline, before handling oxygen cylinders or equipment.
- Never leave oxygen cylinders standing without a stand (even the small E-bottles). They could tip and fall. Oxygen is under high pressure (2,000 psi), and if the cylinder falls and the valve breaks off, the cylinder could act like a rocket due to the high pressure in the bottle.
- Always carry oxygen stand or cart in the car using a bungee cord to anchor it to the back of the seat.
- Always post a sign outside the house entrance that says Oxygen in Use.

Feeding Pump

Precautions on using pump:

- Proper loading or threading of tubing
- Dangerous if feeding rate is too high (causes vomiting, aspirations, diarrhea, etc.)
- If whole amount goes in at once, could cause death
- Position pump so that tubing will not get tangled around the child's neck (a challenge with an active child)

Use right formula in the right amounts (do not rely on measuring marks on the formula bag; use a separate measuring cup.

Ask for the type of bag that contains an ice pouch.

Use an ice bag for overnight feedings to keep formula from souring. Wrap bag with towel to aid in keeping cool longer

Suction Machine

A suction machine is a device that has a compressor that creates a negative pressure vacuum called suction. When tubing is attached, the machine pulls mucus and other secretions up through the catheter and connecting tubing into the collection bottle. There may be a gauge on the machine to indicate how much negative pressure is being created.

Suction machines are available in different models. However, most models have the same basic parts: a regulator knob that allows you to set the proper amount of suction, connecting tubing through which the secretions drain, and a collection bottle that holds the secretions. Some models have a pressure gauge that indicates the amount of suction. Battery operated suction machines also are available.

The suction catheter is placed on the end of the connecting tubing. The catheter has a thumb vent that acts as a control valve. By placing your finger over the vent when the suction machine is on, you can control the amount of suction pressure. The tip of the suction catheter that is placed in the patient's mouth, throat, or in the trach is smooth and has a number of holes to allow mucus and secretions to be pulled into the tubing. A Yankauer catheter may be used for oral suction. For more specific operating instructions, you will need to check with the manual for your suction machine, and you will also receive hands-on instruction from a respiratory therapist.

Proper cleaning and disinfecting of respiratory therapy equipment in the home is very important. It is important to keep your suction machine clean and free from harmful bacteria that could cause an infection.

- Remove the tubing from the outlets on the lid of the collection bottle.
- Remove the lid from the collection bottle.
- Remove the collection bottle from the holder on the suction machine.
- Empty the contents of the collection bottle into the toilet. Do not pour contents in the sink.

- Wash the collection bottle and bottle lid thoroughly in a solution of liquid detergent and warm water. Dry with clean towel.
- Follow your doctors' instructions about cleaning suction catheters. Depending on the patient's condition, you will be using clean technique or sterile technique.
- Make sure when using a suction machine that you replace collection canisters, connecting tubing, and suction catheters that are hard or cracked according to the manufacturers guidelines.

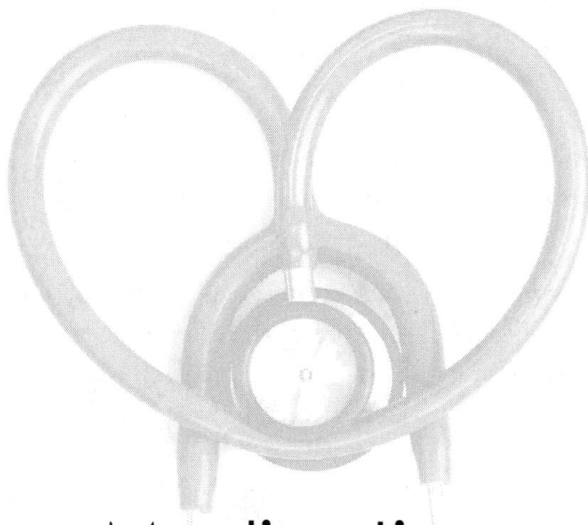

Medication Administration and Required Documentation

Taking Medicine Correctly

For the child's prescription or over-the-counter (OTC) medication to work the way that it should, it is important to follow exact guidelines for its use.

- Stick with the schedule: Prescription medications need to be given consistently and at the right times to help the child get better. Do not skip a dose of the child's medication. When you first get the medication, ask the pediatrician or pharmacist what to do if a dose is not given on time.

- Give the right amount: Measure carefully. Do not be tempted to increase the amount of medication you give the child in an attempt to speed up recovery. Giving the child more medication than is directed may harm him. With both prescription medications and OTCs, follow the directions exactly.
- Know the child's weight: With OTCs, it is best to determine how much medicine to give by checking the label to see how much is recommended for the child's weight. Age is not always an accurate measure of how much medicine the child should receive.
- Do not stop too soon: The child should continue to take his prescription medication for its full course, even if he begins to feel better. The same goes for instances where he does not like the taste of the medication or protests.

You can help prevent overdose or poisoning by following these tips:

- Always use good light. Giving medicine in the dark increases the risk that you will give the wrong medication or the wrong dose.
- Read the label before you open the bottle, after you remove a dose, and again before you give it. This routine can ensure the child's safety.

- Always use child-resistant caps and lock all medications away from the child.
- Give the correct dose. Children are not just small adults. Never guess how much to give the child based on size.
- Do not increase the dose just because the child seems sicker than last time.
- Always follow the weight and age recommendations on the label. If you have questions, ask the pediatrician or call the pharmacy.
- Do not confuse the abbreviations for tablespoon (TBSP or T) and teaspoon (tsp or t).
- Avoid making conversions. If the label calls for two teaspoons and you have a dosing cup labeled only with ounces, do not use it. Use an appropriate measuring device.
- Be sure the pediatrician knows if the child is taking more than one medication at a time.
- Supervise children when they take any medications. Never let young children take medication by themselves.
- Before using any medication, always check for signs of tampering. Do not use any medication from a package that shows cuts, tears, or other imperfections.
- Let your pediatrician know if the child is taking any herbal products, supplements, or home remedies. These substances can interact with many prescription medications and OTCs.

Store your medications in a locked, childproof cabinet that is not located in the bathroom. Medications stored in a bathroom medicine cabinet can be affected by humidity.

It is not always easy to give medication to a child. You may find the infant or toddler hates the taste and spits out the medication or refuses to swallow it. Try adding a little sugar or juice (not honey) to the dosing device to make it taste better. However, do not combine medications with milk or try to mix them into a bowl of cereal. These may affect the medication's active ingredient and limit its absorption. The child also may only eat part of it, or it may settle to the bottom and never get into the mouth.

Older children may be more willing to take chewable tablets than liquid medicines. Although most children's medications are flavored to make them taste better, avoid calling them candy. It might make the toddler decide to take them on his own.

Talk with the pediatrician if you have any questions or concerns about giving the child medications. Keep the pediatrician informed about any changes in how the child is feeling or if the child has any reactions to the medications.

Prescription Medicine

A doctor must order prescription medications. If the child needs a prescription medication, it is very important that you understand the pediatrician and pharmacist's instructions. The following list of questions will help you find out all you need to know:

- What is the name of the medication?
- How will this medication help the child?
- Do I need to do anything before giving this medication to the child?
- How much of the medication do I give the child?
- At what times of the day should I give the medication to the child?
- How long does the child have to take the medication?
- Should the child avoid certain foods or activities while using this medication?
- Should the child avoid other medications, herbal products, or supplements while using this medication?
- Are there any side effects that I should know about?
- Is there anything unusual about how the child is taking this medication (for example, is it a larger than usual dose)?
- Does this medication come in other forms that may be easier for the child to take, such as chewable tablets or liquid?
- Can this prescription be refilled? How many times?
- Is there any written information you can give me?
- What do I do if the child misses a dose?
- What do I do if I give the child too much?

- What if the child spits out the medication?
- Can you show me how to use this medication?

Many medications are available in less expensive forms than brand-name preparations. Often these non-brand-name medications can be used instead of a brand-name medication. Other times, it is more important to use the brand name. Ask the pediatrician if you may use a non-brand-name medication instead of a brand-name medication.

Ask as many questions as you need. If more questions come up after you leave the pediatrician's office, call the office or ask the pharmacist. If the child is old enough, make sure he understands what he must do as well.

Common Over-the-Counter Medications

Over-the-counter (OTC) medications can be bought at your local drugstore or grocery store without a doctor's order. This does not mean that OTCs are harmless. Like prescription medications, OTCs can be very dangerous to a child if taken incorrectly. You need to read and understand the instructions before giving OTCs to the child. The following list describes some common OTCs for children. Talk to the pediatrician before giving any medications to the child. Remember, any child in foster care has to have written prescriptions and instructions for any medications prior to giving the child.

Fever Reducer or Pain Reliever (e.g., acetaminophen, ibuprofen):

If the child has a mild fever but is playing, drinking fluids, and generally acting well, there is no reason to treat the fever. However, if the child complains of headaches, body aches, or seems irritable, there are fever reducers such as acetaminophen and ibuprofen that may help him feel better. They also can help relieve minor pain from bangs and bumps or tenderness from an immunization. Given in the correct dosage, acetaminophen and ibuprofen have few side effects and are quite safe. They come in drops for infants, liquid (elixir) for toddlers, and chewable tablets for older children. Remember, the infant drops are stronger than the liquid elixir for toddlers. Some people make the mistake of giving higher doses of the infant drops to a toddler thinking the drops are not as strong. Be sure the type you give the child is appropriate for his weight and age.

Ibuprofen tends to be more effective than acetaminophen in treating high fevers (103 degrees Fahrenheit or higher). However, ibuprofen should only be given to children older than six months. Never give it to a child who is dehydrated or vomiting continuously. If the child has a kidney disease, asthma, an ulcer, or other chronic illness, ask the pediatrician if it is safe for the child to take ibuprofen. Do not use ibuprofen or acetaminophen with any other pain reliever or fever reducer unless directed by a doctor. Remember, some cold remedies contain these in combination with other medications.

Antihistamines

Antihistamines can relieve runny noses, itchy eyes, and sneezing due to allergies (but not colds). They also relieve itching from chickenpox or insect bites and may even control hives or other allergic reactions. They can make some children sleepy. In other children, they may cause irritability and nervousness, making it difficult for them to rest. For that reason, avoid giving an antihistamine at bedtime until you know it will not make the child have trouble sleeping.

Decongestants

Decongestants can relieve stuffiness due to allergies or colds. However, decongestants taken by mouth can have a number of side effects. Children taking these medications may act hyper, feel anxious, have a racing heart, or find it difficult to sleep. These medications should be used very sparingly.

Nose Drops (Decongestant)

Decongestant nose drops can temporarily shrink the membranes in the nose and make breathing easier. However, they should never be given to an infant because too much of the medication can be absorbed through the membranes of the nose. Also, the more they are used, the less effective they become, and symptoms can return or even get worse. Do not give the child decongestant nose drops for more than two to three days unless the pediatrician advises you to continue this treatment.

Nose Drops (Saltwater/Saline)

Infants and toddlers cannot blow their nose. If the child is sleeping well and eating happily, there is no need to treat the stuffy nose. But if the child is unable to sleep or eat because of thick mucus, saltwater nose drops can help clear the nose. Put a drop or two into a nostril at a time. Using a bulb syringe, squeeze the bulb first, put the tip gently into the child's nostril, and then let go. This will suction out the drops, along with the mucus. Be careful; overuse of a bulb syringe can be irritating to a child's nose.

Cough Syrups

Coughing helps the lungs clear out germs. A cough is productive if it sounds like mucus is being brought up. You can best relieve it by humidifying the air in the child's bedroom to loosen mucus. Be sure to clean the humidifier frequently to prevent mold and bacteria buildup. Some cough medicines, called expectorants, also may help loosen mucus. However, avoid using cough suppressants, as coughing is necessary to clear the lungs. Check with the pediatrician before giving cough medicines or expectorants. Cough syrups may not relieve cough caused by asthma.

Cold Remedies

Combinations of antihistamines and decongestants can have side effects such as hyperactivity, sleeplessness, and irritability. Giving the child more than one cold medicine to treat different symptoms can be dangerous. Many cold medicines contain acetaminophen or ibuprofen. If you are already giving the child acetaminophen or ibuprofen in addition to the cold medicine, this can lead to overdose. Read labels carefully. Check with the pediatrician before giving any cold medicines.

Mild Cortisone Cream

Insect bites, mild skin rashes, poison ivy, or small patches of eczema usually respond to cortisone cream. Never use it for chickenpox, burns, infections, open wounds, or broken skin. Check with the pediatrician before using it repeatedly or using it on the child's face.

Medications Used for Common Gastrointestinal Problems

There are many OTC medications for heartburn, gas, constipation, and diarrhea. Most of these conditions usually go away by themselves or are relieved by a temporary change in diet. Before using any medicine for constipation or diarrhea, talk with the pediatrician. Repeated bouts of diarrhea or chronic constipation can be caused by serious underlying problems.

Using the Correct Dosing Device

Liquid Medications

Many children's medications come in liquid form because they are easier to swallow than pills. But they must be used correctly. Too often people misread the directions, giving children several times the recommended dosage. This can be very dangerous, especially if given over a period of several days. Read the instructions carefully. Call the pediatrician if you are not sure how much, how often, or for how long to give medications to the child. When giving the child a liquid medication, do not use standard tableware tablespoons and teaspoons because they usually are not accurate. Instead, use one of the measuring devices listed below. (Many children's medications come with one. If not, ask the pharmacist for the appropriate dosing device.) These can help you give the right amount of medication.

Syringes and Oral Droppers

These can be very helpful when giving medication to an infant. Simply squirt the medication between the child's tongue and the side of the mouth. This makes it easier for the baby to swallow. Avoid squirting the medicine into the back of the child's throat. This will more likely cause the child to gag and spit the medication out.

Dosing Spoons

These can be useful for older children who will open their mouths and drink from the spoon.

Medication Cups

These often come as caps on liquid cold and flu medications. Make sure to use the cup that comes with the medication. Do not mix and match cups to other products.

Injectable Medications

One cc is equal to one ml (milliliter); the two terms can be used interchangeably. Most syringes are marked cc while medication strengths are marked as milligrams per milliliter (mg/ml). The doctor will calculate just how much medication you will administer with each injection; dosages are calculated based on the strength of the drug and the child's weight and required dose.

One cc syringes have markings showing tenths of a cc: .10 is one-tenth of a cc; 1.0 is one cc; these two measures are frequently confused. Some syringes do not show the decimal point and are marked 10, 20, and 30 on up to 100. In this case, the 10 is one-tenth (.10) of a cc, and the 100 is one cc.

Some 1 cc syringes are further divided, showing markings between the tenths (usually five short lines between the longer tenth lines). There are times when you will be required to administer .05 cc (not to be confused with .5 cc); even without the additional markings between the tenths, half ccs are easily visualized and drawn up. If you are required to pull up something less than a half cc, such as .32, then you would pull up the first small line after the three-tenths (.30) line.

To fill a syringe, begin with the plunger pushed fully down. Insert the needle into the rubber cap of the vial of medication. Hold the vial upside down so that the syringe and needle are pointing toward the ceiling. Gently pull back the plunger to begin the flow of medication into the syringe. Draw slightly more than you need, then push the excess out by pushing the plunger back in; this will get rid of air bubbles that were drawn up from the vial. If you still see air bubbles in the syringe, hold it pointed toward the ceiling and flick or tap your finger against the side of the syringe; this forces the bubbles up toward the hub of the syringe, and you can push the collected air out of the needle. If you need to draw up more medication to make the full dose, stick the needle back into the vial and draw what you need. When you are ready to administer the injection, make sure that the medication is flush up against and into the hub of the syringe. If the medication will not flow into the syringe, you will need to start with some air in the syringe. Before inserting the needle into the bottle of fluid, draw back on the plunger to pull in .5 cc or so of air. After the needle is inserted into the fluid, push down on the plunger to transfer the air in the syringe into the bottle of fluid, then pull back and begin filling your syringe.

Drug Reactions and Interactions

In the event a drug reaction occurs as evidenced by hives, tachypnea, hypertension, hypotension, or any other untoward symptom, the doses and routine should be stopped immediately and the doctor notified. Appropriate drugs will be administered, as ordered, to counteract the reaction.

The administration of medications to children presents a number of problems that are not encountered when giving medication to adult patients. Children vary widely in age, weight, surface area, and the ability to absorb, metabolize, and excrete medications. Foster parents will need to be particularly alert when computing and administering drugs to infants and children.

Always know why you are giving a medication, what the desired effect of the medication is you are giving, and the most common side effects.

Conversion Chart	
.5 ml	½ cc
1 ml	1 cc
¼ teaspoon	1.25 cc
½ teaspoon	2.5 cc
¾ teaspoon	3.75 cc
1 teaspoon	5 cc
½ ounce	15 cc
1 ounce	30 cc
½ cup	120 cc
1 cup	240 cc

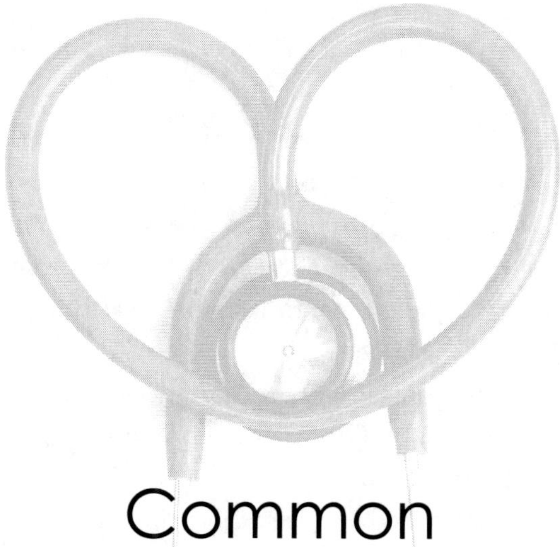

Common Medications and Side Effects

Actigall (Ursodiol): Used for liver disease and helps break down bile. Used commonly with premature infants.

Side effects: side effects are rare, but can sometimes cause abdominal pain, nausea, or vomiting.

Advil, Motrin Drops, Children's Advil, PediaCare Children's Fever (Ibuprofen): Used for mild to moderate pain and lowering of fever.

Side effects: Headache, dizziness, GI bleeding, constipation, nausea, or abdominal discomfort.

Albuterol: Used for asthma or lung disease. Can be ordered routine or as needed. This medication can be ordered orally, as an inhaler, or in a nebulizer.

Side effects: Lightheadedness or fainting, tremors or shaking, or fast, pounding, or irregular heartbeat.

Aldactone (Spironlactone): A diuretic agent that promotes sodium and chloride excretion without concomitant loss of potassium.

Side effects: Fluid and electrolyte imbalance, elevated BUN, Lethargy, mental confusion, fatigue.

Amoxil (Amoxicillin): Treatment of infections, most commonly skin and skin structure infections, otitis media, sinusitis, and respiratory infections.

Side effects: Rashes, diarrhea, nausea, vomiting, urticaria.

Atarax: Used to relieve anxiety, control nausea and emesis. Also used in management of pruritus due to allergic conditions.

Side effects: Drowsiness, sedation, dizziness, headache.

Ativan: Management of anxiety disorders and for short-term relief of symptoms of anxiety. Also used for management of status epilepticus.

Side effects: Drowsiness, sedation, dizziness, sleep disturbance. Usually disappear with continued medication or with reduced dosage.

Atrovent (Ipratropium): Bronchodilator in maintenance therapy of reversible airway obstruction due to COPD, adjunctive management of bronchospasm caused by asthma.

Side effects: Dizziness, headache, nervousness, cough, palpitations, irritation, and nausea.

Baclofen (Lioresal): Treatment of spasticity associated with multiple sclerosis or spinal cord lesions.

Side effects: Dizziness, drowsiness, fatigue, weakness, nausea, constipation.

Bactrim: Antinfective, used for the treatment of infections.

Side effects: Mild to moderate rashes, nausea, vomiting, diarrhea, anorexia.

Bactroban: Used for superficial skin infections.

Side effects: Burning, stinging, pain, pruritus, rash, erythema.

Benadryl: Temporary symptomatic relief of various allergic conditions and to treat or prevent motion sickness, and vertigo. Also used in anaphylaxis as adjunct to epinephrine.

Side effects: Drowsiness, dizziness, headache, palpitations, tinnitus, vertigo.

Captopril (Capoten): Used for management of hypertension, management of left ventricular dysfunction and congestive heart failure.

Side effects: Cough, hypotension, and loss of taste perception.

Carafate (Sucralfate): Used in management of gastric ulcer and maintenance therapy of duodenal ulcers.

Side effects: Constipation, diarrhea, dry mouth, gastric discomfort, indigestion, and rashes.

Cardizem: For treatment of angina and hypertension. Decreases cardiac work, decreases cardiac energy consumption and increases delivery of oxygen to myocardial cells.

Side effects: Dizziness, lightheadedness, peripheral edema, hypotension, flushing, nausea.

Ceclor: Antibiotic used for treatment of a variety of infections such as UTIs, skin infections, and otitis media.

Side effects: Nausea, vomiting, diarrhea, anorexia, rash.

Charcoal: Antidote used for emergency treatment in poisoning by most drugs and chemicals.

Side effects: Vomiting, constipation, diarrhea, black stools.

Cipro (Ciprofloxacin): Treats infections that are caused by bacteria.

Side effects: Allergic reaction such as itching, hives, facial swelling, diarrhea, severe headache, skin rash, vomiting.

Citrate of magnesia: Used for short-term relief of constipation, to prevent straining, to evacuate the bowel for diagnostic procedures.

Side effects: Excessive bowel activity, perianal irritation, abdominal cramps.

Clindamycin: Antibacterial used for serious infections when less toxic alternatives are inappropriate.

Side effects: Diarrhea, abdominal pain, rashes, pruritus, hypotension, generalized myalgia.

Codeine: Used for relief of mild to moderate pain and for suppression of coughing.

Side effects: Sedation, clamminess, sweating, headache, vertigo, floating feeing, dizziness.

Colace: Used prophylactically in patients who should avoid straining during defecation and for treatment of constipation.

Side effects: Occasional mild abdominal cramps, diarrhea, nausea, bitter taste.

Compazine: Control of severe nausea and vomiting.

Side effects: Dry mouth, salivation, nasal congestion, drowsiness, dizziness.

Decadron: Drug has anti-inflammatory and immunosuppression properties. Used to help prevent hyaline membrane disease in premature infants.

Depakote: Used for control of seizures.

Side effects: Sedation, tremor, depression, psychosis, nausea, vomiting.

Desitin: Antidiaper-rash lotion

Side effects: Local irritation, stinging, burning, dermatitis.

Diastat: Used for management of anxiety disorders or for short-term relief of symptoms of anxiety. Also used for severe recurrent seizures.

Side effects: Sedation, depression, lethargy, confusion, slurred speech, stupor, tremor, vertigo.

Dilatin (Phenytoin): Used for seizure control.

Side effects: The most common side effect is drowsiness. This will decrease as the patient becomes used to the medication. This drug can have some serious side effects and labs must be monitored carefully, especially liver.

Epogen: Used for the treatment of anemia.

Side effects: Headache, dizziness, fatigue, nausea, vomiting, diarrhea.

Epsom salt: Used for electrolyte replacement, to control hypertension, and used as laxative.

Side effects: Weakness, dizziness, fainting, sweating, palpitations, excessive bowel activity.

Erthromycin ointment: Used for superficial ocular infections.

Side effects: May cause temporary blurring of vision, stinging, or itching.

Fer-in-sol: Elevates the serum iron concentration.

Side effects: GI upset, anorexia, nausea, vomiting, constipation.

Flagyl (Metronidazole): Treatment for wide range of infections.

Side effects: Dizziness, headache, abdominal pain, anorexia nausea, diarrhea, dry mouth, rashes, vomiting.

Flonase: Used as preventive treatment of asthma, not as primary treatment.

Side effects: Nasal irritation, rash.

Furadantin (Nitrofurantoin): Anti-infective used to treat or prevent infections of the urinary tract. Can also be used to treat other infections.

Side effects: Upset stomach, loss of appetite, vomiting, dizziness, or drowsiness.

Imodium: Used as antidiarrheal, needs prescription. Same drug as Kayexalate.

Side effects: Abdominal pain, distention or discomfort, constipation, dry mouth, nausea, vomiting.

Kayexalate: Used as antidiarrheal. Same drug as Imodium; can be bought over the counter.

Side effects: Abdominal pain, distention or discomfort, constipation, dry mouth, nausea, vomiting.

Keflex: Antibiotic used for bacteria infections.

Side effects: Nausea, vomiting, diarrhea, anorexia, abdominal pain.

Keppra (Levetiracetam): Used for seizure control.

Side effects: extreme sleepiness, tiredness, weakness or problems with muscle coordination.

Ketoconazole: Used for treatment of fungal infections.

Side effects: Nausea, headache, dizziness, vomiting. With local application, severe irritation, stinging, and pruritus.

Klonopin: Used for treatment of seizures.

Side effects: Sedation, depression, lethargy, fatigue, restlessness, constipation, diarrhea, dry mouth, hiccups.

Lactulase: Used as laxative and prevention and treatment of portal-systemic encephalopathy.

Side effects: Transient flatulence, distention, intestinal cramps, diarrhea, nausea.

Lanoxin (Digoxin): widely used cardiac drug, acts by increasing the force and velocity of contraction.

Side effects: Fatigue, muscle weakness, headache, drowsiness, nausea, and diaphoresis.

Lasix (Furosemide): Used for treatment of edema associated with CHF, cirrhosis of liver, and kidney disease. May be used for management of hypertension.

Side effects: Hypovolemia, dehydration, hyponatremia, nausea, vomiting.

Lomotil: Used for treatment of diarrhea.

Side effects: Abdominal pain, cramps, nausea, abdominal distention.

Maalox: Used as antiflatulent.

Side effects: Nausea, vomiting, diarrhea, constipation, belching, passing of flatus.

Methadone: Used for relief of severe pain. Also used for detoxification and temporary maintenance treatment of opioid addiction.

Side effects: Respiratory depression, nausea, lightheadedness, facial flushing, vomiting, sweating.

Nasonex: Used for relief of inflammatory and pruritic manifestations of corticosteroid-sensitive dermatoses.

Side effects: Burning, irritation, skin atrophy, secondary infection.

Norvasc (Amlodipine): Used to control high blood pressure or angina.

Side effects: Nausea, fatigue, weakness, stomach pain, muscle cramps, headache, or flushing.

Nystatin: Antifungal used for treatment of oropharyngeal candidiasis (oral form), topical application is used for local treatment of vaginal candidiasis.

Side effects: Nausea, vomiting, diarrhea with oral form, local irritation and burning.

Orapred: Short-term management of various inflammatory and allergic disorders.

Side effects: Immunosuppression, or masking of infections, vertigo, headache, depression, increased appetite, weight gain.

Pepcid (Famotidine): Used for treatment of GI reflex or gastroesophageal reflux disease (GERD).

Side effects: Side effects of famotidine are rare. Minor side effects include constipation, diarrhea, fatigue, headache, insomnia, muscle pain, nausea, and vomiting.

Phenergan (Promethazine): Treatment of various allergic conditions and motion sickness, treatment for prevention of nausea and vomiting.

Side effects: Sedation, dizziness, fatigue, nervousness, and rashes.

Phenobarbital: Used for seizure control, and sometimes used for infants with severe drug withdrawals.

Side effects: The most common side effect is drowsiness. This can be temporary, but will return each time the dose is increased. A rare side effect is a body rash.

Prednisone: Used as anti-inflammatory.

Side effects: Headache, insomnia, confusion, delayed wound healing.

Prevacid (Lansoprazole): Used for short-term treatment of symptomatic GERD, management of duodenal ulcers.

Side effects: Dizziness, headache, diarrhea, abdominal pain, nausea, rash.

Prilosec: Suppresses gastric acid secretion, relieving gastrointestinal distress and promoting ulcer healing.

Side effects: Diarrhea, abdominal pain, nausea, rash.

Protopic: Used for liver rejection prophylaxis, rejection prophylaxis for other organ transplants, and moderate to severe atopic dermatitis.

Side effects: Headache, tremors, nausea, abdominal pain, gas, appetite changes.

Pseudophedrine: Used for temporary relief of nasal congestion caused by the common cold, hay fever, other respiratory allergies.

Side effects: CNS depression, weakness, seizures, nausea, vomiting, hypertension.

Pulmicort (Budesonide): Used to prevent asthma attacks. Not effective for acute attack.

Side effects: Allergic reaction such as hives, swelling of face or hands, sore throat, runny nose, tingling in the month.

Reglan (Metoclopramide): Used for management of esophageal reflux, also used for postoperative nausea and vomiting.

Side effects: Drowsiness, restlessness, anxiety, depression, and irritability.

Respiratory Syncytial Virus Immune Globulin (RSV IG) injectable: Used for prevention of serious lower respiratory tract infection caused by RSV in children less twenty-four months with bronchopulmonary dysplasia or history of premature birth.

Side effects: Must have epinephrine 1:1000 available for first dose at time of injection in case of anaphylactic reaction, discomfort at injection site.

Risperdal: Used for the treatment of schizophrenia and treatment of irritability, aggression, self-injury, temper tantrums, quickly changing moods.

Side effects: Insomnia, anxiety, headache, orthostatic hypotension, nausea, vomiting, dry mouth.

Ritalin: Used for treatment of attention-deficit disorders, hyperkinetic syndrome, minimal brain dysfunction in children.

Side effects: Nervousness, insomnia, dizziness, rash, urticaria, anorexia, nausea, abdominal pain, weight loss.

Robinul: Used for the reduction of salivary, tracheobronchial, and pharyngeal secretions, reduction of the volume and free acidity of gastric secretions.

Side effects: Dry mouth, altered taste perception, nausea, vomiting, urinary hesitancy and retention.

Robitussin: Symptomatic relief of respiratory conditions characterized by dry, nonproductive cough and when there is mucus in the respiratory tract.

Side effects: Nausea, vomiting, dizziness, headache, rash, GI discomfort.

Rocephin: Antibiotic used for a variety of different bactericidal infections.

Side effects: Nausea, vomiting, diarrhea, anorexia, abdominal pain, hepatotoxicity, flatulence.

Senokot: Used for short-term relief of constipation to prevent straining.

Side effects: Excessive bowel activity, abdominal cramps, weakness, dizziness, dependence.

Singulair: Used for prophylaxis and chronic treatment for asthma, relief of symptoms of seasonal allergic rhinitis.

Side effects: Headache, dizziness, nausea, vomiting, dental pain.

Solu-Medrol: Short-term management of various inflammatory and allergic disorders, such as rheumatoid arthritis, collagen diseases, dermatologic diseases, status asthmaticus, and autoimmune disorders.

Side effects: Vertigo, headache, increased appetite, weight gain, immunosuppression, masking of infections, impaired wound healing, thin, fragile skin, and glaucoma.

Tagamet (Cimetidine): Used for management of gastroesophageal reflux disease (GERD), heartburn, acid indigestion, and sour stomach.

Side effects: Dizziness, drowsiness, constipation, diarrhea, nausea.

Tegretol: Used for the treatment of seizures, tic douloureux, and treatment of acute manic and mixed episodes associated with bipolar disorders.

Side effects: Dizziness, drowsiness, unsteadiness, photosensitivity reactions, nausea, vomiting, gastric distress, liver damage.

Tetracycline: Antibiotic used for a variety of infections.

Side effects: Discoloring and inadequate calcification of primary teeth of fetus if used by pregnant women, discoloring and inadequate calcification of permanent teeth if used during period of dental development. Also nausea, vomiting, diarrhea, glossitis, dysphagia.

Theophyline: Used as bronchial widener. It is given to relax the smooth muscle of the bronchial passages in the treatment of bronchospasm in bronchial asthma, bronchitis, and emphysema. Not to be used with history of high blood pressure, heart disease, liver disease, kidney disease, or simultaneous treatment with other xanthines prohibits its use.

Side effects: Most common is palpitations and agitation. Among the most serious side effects are allergy, bleeding in the stomach and intestines, palpitations, and seizures.

Tigan: Used for control of nausea and vomiting.

Side effects: Parkinsonlike symptoms, dizziness, drowsiness, headache, allergic-type skin reactions.

Tinactin: Used as topical antifungal.

Side effects: Local irritation, stinging, burning, dermatitis.

Tobramycin (Tobramycin): Inhalant, helps treat pseudomonas infections.

Side effects: Increased coughing, wheezing, ringing in ears, skin rash.

Topamax (Topiramate): Used for treatment of seizures.

Side effects: Dizziness, drowsiness, fatigue, abnormal vision, nausea, abdominal pain, ataxia, constipation, dry mouth.

Valium (Diazepam): Treatment for uncontrolled seizures, skeletal muscle relaxant, and management of the symptoms of alcohol withdrawal.

Side effects: Dizziness, drowsiness, lethargy, depression, blurred vision, respiratory depression.

Valproic Acid: Used for treatment of seizures.

Side effects: Sedation, tremor, nausea, vomiting, indigestion, pancreatitis, liver damage, weakness.

Vancomycin: Antibiotic used for potentially life-threatening infections not treatable with other less toxic antibiotics.

Side effects: Ototoxicity, hypotension, urticaria, nausea, nephrotoxicity.

Xopenex: Treatment or prevention of bronchospasm in patients with reversible obstructive airway disease.

Side effects: Migraine, dizziness, nervousness, tremor, anxiety

Zantac (Ranitidine): Used for management of Gastroesophageal reflux disease (GERD), treatment of heartburn, acid indigestion, and sour stomach.

Side effects: Dizziness, drowsiness, confusion, constipation, diarrhea, nausea, and anemia.

Zeasorb: Topical antifungal.

Side effects: Irritation, sensitization, rash, headache.

Zinc: Dietary supplement to treat or prevent zinc deficiencies.

Side effects: Vomiting, nausea.

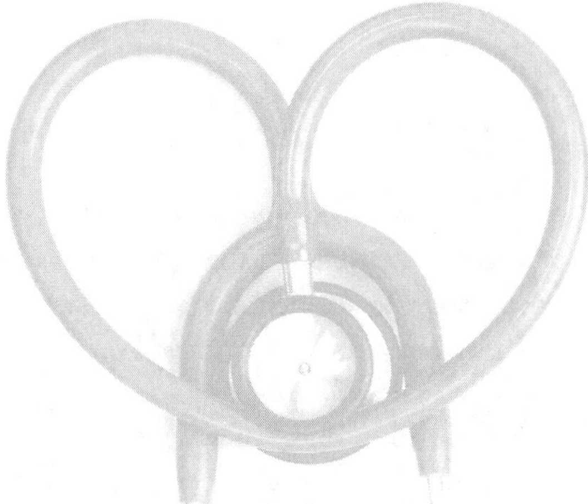

Common Medical Surgeries and Tests

Anesthesia

Anesthesia is the loss of sensitivity to pain brought about by various drugs (anesthetics). Anesthesia is used during many medical procedures, including surgical procedures. The type of anesthesia that the child will receive depends on the procedure being performed and the physical and emotional status of the child. Knowing the type of anesthesia that the child will receive before a medical procedure or surgery will help you know what to expect in terms of preparation, pain relief, and recovery.

Types of Anesthesia

Anesthesia can be categorized by the degree to which it suppresses consciousness and protective reflexes. Larger procedures often require greater amounts of anesthesia. From least to most, levels of anesthesia include: local, conscious sedation, regional, and general. Determining the best choice for the child depends on the anticipated nature and duration of the procedure, as well as medical health.

Local Anesthesia

Local anesthesia is used to block pain in a specific part of the body, allowing the patient to remain fully alert. The area that is anesthetized is usually small and superficial. Typically, a local anesthetic is used for dental work, skin biopsies, or stitching up a cut. Sometimes a local anesthetic is used for a more extensive procedure in people for whom general or regional anesthesia is inadvisable. For local anesthesia, an anesthetic is injected at or near the site of the procedure. The injection numbs the area to pain and any other sensation. Local anesthetics are generally of short duration. They come in different forms, including injections, sprays, and ointments. Only rarely do they cause an allergic reaction.

Conscious Sedation

Conscious sedation or intravenous (IV) sedation is used to relax the patient and make them feel sleepy. It generally includes intravenous administration of pain medication and a mild sedative to minimize any discomfort. These medications also cause temporary forgetfulness, so the patient may not remember what happens during the procedure. Even though the patient may not remember anything that occurs during conscious sedation, they remain awake enough during that time to respond to questions and retain their protective reflexes. For example, if secretions accumulated in the throat, the patient would swallow or cough. This type of anesthesia is used for procedures such as colonoscopy, an exam of the colon and rectum. Conscious sedation is also frequently combined with regional anesthesia.

Regional Anesthesia

Regional anesthesia is used to block sensation in a particular region of the body, such as the lower half of the body, an eye, an arm, or leg. As with local anesthesia, the patient will remain conscious during regional anesthesia. Often, regional anesthesia is combined with conscious sedation, so the patient might not remember any of the procedure. The anesthetic is injected around a single nerve or a network of nerves that serve the area involved in the surgical procedure. The patient will receive the injection, which is generally painless, while lying on their back or side or sitting. To eliminate pain in the lower half of the body, spinal, epidural, or caudal anesthetics may be injected near the spinal cord. These forms of anesthesia are often used for pelvic operations and for leg and hip surgery. Epidural anesthesia is often used during childbirth. The main advantage of regional anesthesia is that it provides a high level of anesthesia to a selected region of the body while having little effect on other areas, such as the heart, lungs, and brain. In regional anesthesia, the protective reflexes remain intact. An additional benefit of regional anesthesia is that it helps control post-operative pain. That means the patient may require less pain medication after surgery and can avoid the nausea and grogginess that often result from those medications.

General Anesthesia

General anesthesia is used for more extensive procedures or for procedures that aren't amenable to regional anesthesia. The medications used in general anesthesia are given intravenously or by inhalation. The drugs circulate in the bloodstream to all areas of the body, including the brain. They can suppress all of the protective reflexes, such as coughing, gagging, and even breathing. Consequently, a general anesthetic requires the use of a mask or breathing tube while the patient is asleep.

Because general anesthetics affect all areas of the body, such as the heart and lungs, side effects from the medications are more common. However, most are temporary and can be managed by the medical team.

Cardiac Catheterization

During this procedure, a long, thin tube called a catheter is threaded through blood vessels in the navel (in a newborn) or the groin and up into the heart. Once in place, the catheter can measure the oxygen levels and pressures within the heart's chambers. Dye may be injected through the catheter to better illustrate the heart's inner structures and determine the direction of blood flow through the heart. Certain defects can be fixed in the cardiac catheterization laboratory. For instance, there are devices that can be used to close holes in the heart.

Computerized Axial Tomography Scan (CAT Scan)

A computerized axial tomography scan is more commonly known by its abbreviated name, CAT scan or CT scan. It is an X-ray procedure that combines many X-ray images with the aid of a computer to generate cross-sectional views and, if needed, three-dimensional images of the internal organs and structures of the body. A CAT scan is used to define normal and abnormal structures in the body and/or assist in procedures by helping to accurately guide the placement of instruments or treatments. A large donut-shaped X-ray machine takes X-ray images at many different angles around the body. These images are processed by a computer to produce cross-sectional pictures of the body. In each of these pictures the body is seen as an X-ray slice of the body, which is recorded on a film. This recorded image is called a tomogram. Computerized axial tomography refers to the recorded tomogram sections at different levels of the body.

Imagine the body as a loaf of bread, and you are looking at one end of the loaf. As you remove each slice of bread, you can see the entire surface of that slice from the crust to the center. The body is seen on CAT scan slices in a similar fashion from the skin to the central part of the body being examined. When these levels are further added together, a three-dimensional picture of an organ or abnormal body structure can be obtained.

CAT scans are performed to analyze the internal structures of various parts of the body. This includes the head, where traumatic injuries, (such as blood clots or skull fractures), tumors, and infections can be identified. In the spine, the bony structure of the vertebrae can be accurately defined, as can the anatomy of the intervertebral discs and spinal cord. In fact, CAT scan methods can be used to accurately measure the density of bone in evaluating osteoporosis.

Occasionally, contrast material (an X-ray dye) is placed into the spinal fluid to further enhance the scan and the various structural relationships of the spine, the spinal cord, and its nerves. CAT scans are also used in the chest to identify tumors, cysts, or infections that may be suspected on a chest X-ray. CAT scans of the abdomen are extremely helpful in defining body organ anatomy, including visualizing the liver, gallbladder, pancreas, spleen, aorta, kidneys, uterus, and ovaries. CAT scans in this area are used to verify the presence or absence of tumors, infection, abnormal anatomy, or changes of the body from trauma.

The technique is painless and can provide extremely accurate images of body structures, in addition to guiding the radiologist in performing certain procedures, such as biopsies of suspected cancers, removal of internal body fluids for various tests, and the draining of abscesses that are deep in the body. Many of these procedures are minimally invasive and have a markedly decreased the need to perform surgery to accomplish the same goal.

A CAT scan is a very low-risk procedure. The most common problem is an adverse reaction to intravenous contrast material. Intravenous contrast is usually an iodine-based liquid given in the vein, which makes many organs and structures, such as the kidneys and blood vessels much more visible on the CAT scan. There may be resulting itching, a rash, hives, or a feeling of warmth throughout the body. These are usually self-limiting reactions and go away rather quickly. If needed, antihistamines can be given to help relieve the symptoms. A more serious reaction to intravenous contrast is called an anaphylactic reaction. When this occurs, the patient may experience severe hives and/or extreme difficulty in breathing. This reaction is quite rare, but is potentially life threatening if not treated.

Medications that include corticosteroids, antihistamines, and epinephrine reverse this adverse reaction.

Toxicity to the kidneys that can result in kidney failure is an extremely rare complication of the intravenous contrast used in CAT scans. Diabetics, dehydrated individuals, or patients who already have impaired kidney function are most prone to this reaction. The amount of radiation a person receives during a CAT scan is minimal. In preparation for a CAT scan, patients are often asked to avoid food, especially when contrast material is to be used. Contrast material may be injected intravenously or administered by mouth or by an enema in order to increase the distinction between various organs or areas of the body. Therefore, fluids and food may be restricted for several hours prior to the examination. If the patient has a history of allergy to contrast material (such as iodine), the physician and radiology staff should be notified. All metallic materials and certain clothing around the body are removed because they can interfere with the clarity of the images.

Patients are placed on a movable table, and the table is slipped into the center of a large donut-shaped machine that takes the X-ray images around the body. The actual procedure can take from a half an hour to an hour and a half. If specific tests, biopsies, or intervention are performed by the radiologist during CAT scanning, additional time and monitoring may be required. It is important during the CAT scan procedure that the patient minimizes any body movement by remaining as still and quiet as is possible. This significantly increases the clarity of the X-ray images. The CAT scan technologist tells the patient when to breathe or hold his or her breathe during scans of the chest and abdomen. If any problems are experienced during the CAT scan, the technologist should be informed immediately. The technologist directly watches the patient through an observation window during the procedure, and there is an intercom system in the room for added patient safety.

CAT scans have vastly improved the ability of doctors to diagnose many diseases earlier in their course and with much less risk than previous methods.

CAT Scan Summary

- CAT scanning adds X-ray images with the aid of a computer to generate cross-sectional views of anatomy.
- CAT scanning can identify normal and abnormal structures and be used to guide procedures.
- CAT scanning is painless.
- Iodine-containing contrast material is sometimes used in CAT scanning. Patients with a history of allergy to iodine or contrast materials should notify their physicians and radiology staff.

Magnetic Resonance Imaging Scan (MRI Scan)

An MRI (or magnetic resonance imaging) scan is a radiology technique that uses magnetism, radio waves, and a computer to produce images of body structures. The MRI scanner is a tube surrounded by a giant circular magnet.

The patient is placed on a moveable bed that is inserted into the magnet. The magnet creates a strong magnetic field that aligns the protons of hydrogen atoms, which are then exposed to a beam of radio waves. This spins the various protons of the body, and they produce a faint signal that is detected by the receiver portion of the MRI scanner. The receiver information is processed by a computer, and an image is produced.

The image and resolution produced by MRI is quite detailed and can detect tiny changes of structures within the body. For some procedures, contrast agents are used to increase the accuracy of the images.

An MRI scan can be used as an extremely accurate method of disease detection throughout the body. In the head, trauma to the brain can be seen as bleeding or swelling. Other abnormalities often found include brain aneurysms, stroke, tumors of the brain, as well as tumors or inflammation of the spine. Neurosurgeons use an MRI scan not only in defining brain anatomy but also in evaluating the integrity of the spinal cord after trauma. It is also used when considering problems associated with the vertebrae or intervertebral discs of the spine. An MRI scan can evaluate the structure of the heart and aorta, where it can detect aneurysms or tears. It provides valuable information on glands and organs within the abdomen and accurate information about the structure of the joints, soft tissues, and bones of the body. Often, surgery can be deferred or more accurately directed after knowing the results of an MRI scan.

An MRI scan is a painless radiology technique that

has the advantage of avoiding X-ray radiation exposure. There are no known side effects of an MRI scan. The benefits of an MRI scan relate to its precise accuracy in detecting structural abnormalities of the body. Patients who have any metallic materials within the body must notify their physician prior to the examination or inform the MRI staff. Metallic chips, materials, surgical clips, or foreign material (artificial joints, metallic bone plates, or prosthetic devices, etc.) can significantly distort the images obtained by the MRI scanner. Patients who have heart pacemakers, metal implants, or metal chips or clips in or around the eyeballs cannot be scanned with an MRI because of the risk that the magnet may move the metal in these areas. Similarly, patients with artificial heart valves, metallic ear implants, bullet fragments, and chemotherapy or insulin pumps should not have MRI scanning.

During the MRI scan, patients lie in a closed area inside the magnetic tube. Some patients can experience a claustrophobic sensation during the procedure. Therefore, patients with any history of claustrophobia should relate this to the radiology staff. A mild sedative can be given prior to the MRI scan to help alleviate this feeling. It is customary that the MRI staff will be nearby during MRI scan. Furthermore, there is usually a means of communication with the staff (such as a buzzer held by the patient) that can be used for contact if the patient cannot tolerate the scan.

MRI scanning requires that the patient lie still for best accuracy. Patients lie within a closed environment inside the magnetic machine. Relaxation is important during the procedure, and patients are asked to breathe normally.

Interaction with the MRI technologist is maintained throughout the test. There are loud, repetitive clicking noises that occur during the test as the scanning proceeds. Occasionally, patients require injections of liquid intravenously to enhance the images that are obtained. The MRI scanning time depends on the exact area of the body studied, but ranges from half an hour to an hour and a half.

Nissen Fundoplication

Also referred to as the wrap or fundo, a surgery called the Nissen fundoplication is the final option for controlling very severe gastroesophageal reflux disease. Because of the possible complications that can accompany this surgery, it is typically done as a last resort. It is by no means a cure for GERD and is only performed when severe symptoms and complications persist. It involves wrapping the upper portion of the stomach (fundus) around the lower portion of the esophagus. There are different types of fundus performed. The Nissen fundoplication refers to wrapping the fundus all the way (360 degrees) around the esophagus.

Gastroesophageal reflux disease (GERD) is a digestive disorder that affects the lower esophageal sphincter (LES), the muscle connecting the esophagus with the stomach. Many people, including pregnant women, suffer from heartburn or acid indigestion caused by GERD. Doctors believe that some people suffer from GERD due to a condition called hiatal hernia. In most cases, heartburn can be relieved through diet and lifestyle changes; however, some people may require medication or surgery.

Gastroesophageal refers to the stomach and esophagus. Reflux means to flow back or return. Therefore, gastroesophageal reflux is the return of the stomach's contents back up into the esophagus. In normal digestion, the lower esophageal sphincter opens to allow food to pass into the stomach and closes to prevent food and acidic stomach juices from flowing back into the esophagus. Gastroesophageal reflux occurs when the lower esophageal sphincter is weak or relaxes inappropriately, allowing the stomach's contents to flow up into the esophagus. The severity of GERD depends on lower esophageal sphincter dysfunction as well as the type and amount of fluid brought up from the stomach and the neutralizing effect of saliva.

Fundoplication surgery can be performed as an open procedure or a laparoscopic procedure. The operation is basically the same, but the way the surgeon gets to the stomach and esophagus is different. A laparoscopic fundoplication means that the surgeon will use several small incisions and special instruments with the aid of a videoscope and TV monitors to perform the fundoplication. The recovery time from a laparoscopic fundoplication is shorter than the open procedure. There is also less post-operative pain and a less visible scar. Not all fundoplications can be done laparoscopically because of adhesions from previous operations, excessive bleeding obscuring vision, too much fatty tissue, or other problems; in this case, the standard method called an open fundo would be required.

The patient is put under general anesthesia. In the laparoscopic method, five tiny incisions are made in the abdomen; if the method being used is open, one much larger incision is made. With the laparoscopic method, one incision is used for the laparoscope and the other four are used to insert special devices with which to perform the surgery. Many surgeons will perform gastronomy at the time of the fundo to place a g-tube. The decision to place the g-tube is made based on the surgeon's preferences, medical condition, the child's age, and eating habits prior to surgery. This will likely be in place for a few months to assist with feeding and gas bloat problems. Some children may require the g-tube be in place longer than that.

When the fundo is completed successfully, it works by keeping the lower esophageal sphincter closed enough to prevent reflux while still allowing food to pass through the esophagus and into the stomach.

Orchiopexy

Surgery to move an undescended testicle into the scrotum is called orchiopexy or orchidopexy. It is usually performed on infants and young boys between age six months and one year. It is usually performed by a pediatric surgeon or a specialist who treats urinary problems in children (pediatric urologist).

Orchiopexy may also be done on older boys and, rarely, teens and adult men with undescended testicles. It is usually recommended that an untreated undescended testicle in adult men and teens after puberty be removed rather than moved to the scrotum because of the increased risk of testicular cancer.

Depending on the location of the testicle, one or two

small openings are made in the scrotum, the groin, or the abdomen to allow the surgeon to reach the testicle and move it to the scrotum. Sometimes a surgical method called laparoscopy is used to move undescended testicles when they are located high in the inguinal canal or in the abdomen. In both types of orchiopexy, general anesthesia is used.

Most orchiopexies can be completed in a single operation; however, in some cases when the testicles are located in the abdomen, the surgery may need to be done in two steps with separate operations several months apart. In some cases, an undescended testicle must be removed from the body entirely and then reimplanted in the scrotum (testicular autotransplantation) and the surrounding tissues and blood vessels reattached.

Ultrasound

An ultrasound test is a radiology technique that uses high-frequency sound waves to produce images of the organs and structures of the body. The sound waves are sent through body tissues with a device called a transducer. The transducer is placed directly on top of the skin, which has a gel applied to the surface. The sound waves that are sent by the transducer through the body are then reflected by internal structures as echoes. These echoes return to the transducer and are transmitted electrically onto a viewing monitor. The echo images are then recorded on a plane film and can also be recorded on videotape. After the ultrasound, the gel is easily wiped off. The technical term for ultrasound testing and recording is sonography. Ultrasound testing is painless and harmless. Ultrasound tests involve no radiation and studies have not revealed any adverse effects.

Ultrasound examinations can be used in various areas of the body for a variety of purposes. These purposes include examination of the chest, abdomen, blood vessels (such as to detect blood clots in leg veins) and the evaluation of pregnancy. In the chest, ultrasound can be used to obtain detailed images of the size and function of the heart. An ultrasound can detect abnormalities of the heart valves, such as mitral valve prolapse, aortic stenosis, and infection (endocarditis). An ultrasound is commonly used to guide fluid withdrawal (aspiration) from the chest, lungs, or around the heart. Ultrasounds are also commonly used to examine internal structures of the abdomen. Gallstones in the gallbladder are easily detected, as are kidney stones. The size and structure of the kidneys, the ureters, liver, spleen, pancreas, and aorta within the abdomen can be examined. An ultrasound can detect fluid, cysts, tumors, or abscess in the abdomen or liver. Impaired blood flow from clots or arteriosclerosis in the legs can be detected by ultrasound. Aneurysms of the aorta can also be seen. Ultrasounds are also commonly used to evaluate the structure of the thyroid gland in the neck.

During pregnancy, an ultrasound can be used to evaluate the size, gender, movement, and position of the growing baby. The baby's heart is usually visible early, and as the baby ages, body motion becomes more apparent. The baby can often be visualized by the mother during the ultrasound, and the gender of the baby is sometimes detectable.

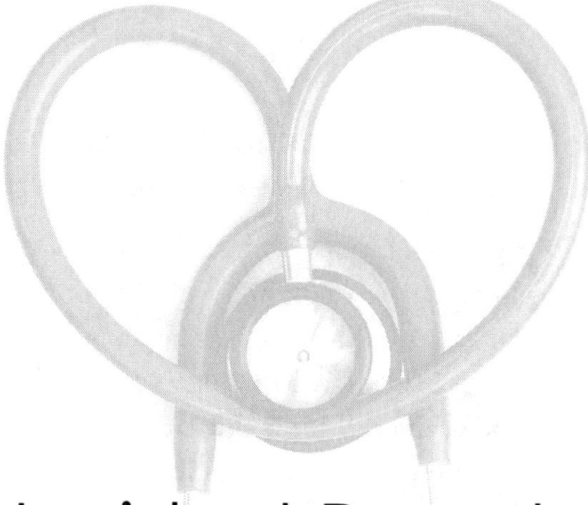

Incident Reports and Why They Are Necessary

Incident reports are very important. Not only does licensing or your agency require them, they are for your protection! Along with all your other documentation from the doctors and medical reports, if this child is frequently ill, even with the best of care, the incident reports will provide this documentation. Any time that the child requires hospitalization or is transported by ambulance or receives any emergency treatment, you must file an incident report. (See sample form.) Provide as much information as possible and be as thorough as possible to events that lead up to the incident and actions taken.

What to do when a baby or child dies under your care in your home

At some time, you may have a child who dies under your care. If this unfortunate event happens in your home, you will call 911 and start CPR as soon as possible. If the paramedics decide that CPR is to be discontinued, then the coroner will be notified. This is the time that you have to remind yourself that all questions and the following investigation is to protect you, and the child deserves the right to have the death thoroughly investigated. Law enforcement will make a separate investigation, then licensing.

If a child dies under your care in the hospital setting

In this situation, you will also be investigated by all the same agencies as if the child had died at your home. It is viewed that the child received care from you prior to the hospitalization, so, again, documentation is very important, and it is for your protection!

Whom to call and when

You will need to notify community care licensing, the child's social worker, and the regional center as soon as possible. If it is during the weekend or holiday, you will be given a 1–800 number that can be used. It may be best to have the social worker tell the parents if needed.

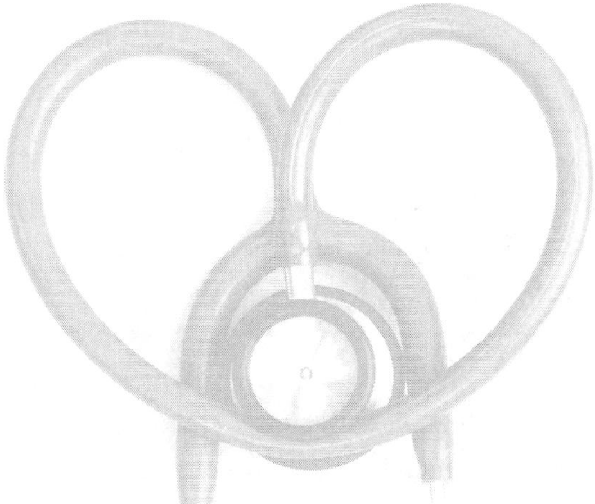

What is CCS and How to Use It

CCS (California Children's Services) is a statewide program that treats children with certain physical limitations and chronic health conditions or diseases. CCS can authorize and pay for specific medical services and equipment provided by CCS-approved specialists. The California Department of Health Services manages the CCS program. Larger counties operate their own CCS programs, while smaller counties share the operation of their program with state CCS regional offices in Sacramento, San Francisco, and Los Angeles. The program is funded with state, county, and federal tax monies, along with some fees paid by parents.

If you or the child's doctor thinks that the child might have a CCS-eligible medical condition, CCS may pay for or provide a medical evaluation to find out if the child's condition is covered.

If the child is eligible, CCS may pay for or provide the following:

Treatment such as doctor services, hospital and surgical care, physical therapy and occupational therapy, laboratory tests, X-rays, orthopedic appliances, and medical equipment

Medical case management to help get special doctors and care for your child when medically necessary and referral to other agencies, including public health nursing and regional centers, or a medical therapy program (MTP), which can provide physical therapy and/or occupational therapy in public schools for children who are medically eligible.

The program is open to anyone who:

- Is under twenty-one years old
- Has or may have a medical condition that is covered by CCS
- Is a resident of California
- Has a family income of $40,000 or less as reported as the adjusted gross income on the state tax form or the out-of-pocket medical expenses for a child who qualifies are expected to be more than 20 percent of family income or the child has Healthy Families coverage

Family income is not a factor for children who:

- Need diagnostic services to confirm a CCS eligible medical condition
- Were adopted with a known CCS-eligible medical condition
- Are applying only for services through the medical therapy program
- Are Medi-Cal beneficiaries, full scope, no share of cost
- Are Healthy Families subscribers

Only certain conditions are covered by CCS. In general, CCS covers medical conditions that are physically disabling or require medical, surgical, or rehabilitative services. There also may be certain criteria that determine if the child's medical condition is eligible. Listed below are categories of medical conditions that may be covered and some examples of each:

- Conditions involving the heart (congenital heart disease)
- Neoplasms (cancers, tumors)
- Disorders of the blood (hemophilia, sickle cell anemia)
- Endocrine, nutritional, and metabolic diseases (thyroid problems, PKU, diabetes)
- Disorders of the genito-urinary system (serious chronic kidney problems)
- Disorders of the gastrointestinal system (chronic inflammatory disease, diseases of the liver)

- Serious birth defects (cleft lip/palate, spina bifida)
- Disorders of the sense organs (hearing loss, glaucoma, cataracts)
- Disorders of the nervous system (cerebral palsy, uncontrolled seizures)
- Disorders of the musculoskeletal system and connective tissues (rheumatoid arthritis, muscular dystrophy)
- Severe disorders of the immune system (HIV infection)
- Disabling conditions or poisonings requiring intensive care or rehabilitation (severe head, brain, or spinal cord injuries, severe burns)
- Complications of premature birth requiring an intensive level of care
- Disorders of the skin and subcutaneous tissue (severe hemangioma)
- Medically handicapping malocclusion (severely crooked teeth)

For more information on medical eligibility, please read this overview or contact your county CCS office. Families (or the applicant if age eighteen or older or an emancipated minor) must:

- Complete an application form (in English or Spanish) and return it to their county CCS office

- Give CCS all of the information requested so CCS can determine if the family qualifies
- Apply to Medi-Cal if CCS believes that a family's income qualifies them for the Medi-Cal program. (If a family qualifies for Medi-Cal, the child is also covered by CCS. CCS approves the services; payment is made through Medi-Cal.)
- For foster children, you are not required to fill out the personal income portions of the form. As the foster mother or father, you are not permitted to sign. The application must be signed by the child's social worker.

The MTP is a special program within California Children's Services that includes occupational therapy (OT) and physical therapy (PT) for children with eligible conditions. Therapy services are provided at rehabilitation units located in public schools. These units are called medical therapy units (MTU).

Eligible conditions that would qualify for CCS and the MTP include, but are not limited to, cerebral palsy, spina bifida, muscular dystrophy, rheumatoid arthritis, spinal cord injuries, arthrogryposis, and osteogenesis imperfecta. For more information on medical eligibility for the MTP, please refer to California Code of Regulations (Title 22, Division 2, Part 2, Subdivision 7, CCS, Chapter 4, Medical Therapy Program, Section 41832).

The MTP is available to children from birth to twenty-one years old with eligible conditions. Just like the general

CCS program, anyone, such as a parent, teacher, school nurse, or physician can refer a child to the MTP.

When the child has been determined medically eligible for the MTP, which requires review of the child's medical record, the child is referred to the local MTU for a therapy evaluation.

A physician is always required for the management of the child's therapy needs and prescriptions in conjunction with the OT and PT evaluations. Evaluations are completed on the child and reviewed with the physician and parents to develop a medical therapy plan tailored to the child's specific therapy needs. OT and/or PT is approved and prescribed by the physician and are provided at the MTU.

Occupational therapy (OT) is therapy provided for the main purpose of improving self-help skills or activities of daily living (ADL). OT uses many ways to improve the dysfunction that causes impairment in ADLs, such as playing with play dough to increase finger strength to allow a child to be able to manage pants snaps. The therapy is provided by a trained occupational therapist that has at least received a bachelor degree, graduated from an approved school of occupational therapy, and has a license from the state of California to provide occupational therapy.

Physical Therapy (PT) is therapy provided for the main purpose of improving mobility and ambulation. PT may provide exercises on a large ball to increase trunk control and overall strength to allow a child to walk either unassisted or with crutches. The therapy is provided by a trained physical therapist that has at least received a bachelor degree, graduated from an approved school of physical therapy, and has a license from the state of California to provide physical therapy.

Periodic evaluations are completed by the MTP team consisting of the physician, OT, and PT and are discussed with the parents. Home exercise programs and home evaluations are conducted by OT and PT to assess accessibility and adaptive equipment needs. Meetings are held with parents and child and rehabilitation equipment specialists to obtain appropriate specialized equipment such as wheelchairs, bathroom equipment, and braces.

MTP therapy staff attends individualized educational plan (IEP) meetings to represent the medical therapy services need of the child and to make sure school personnel are aware of the services provided by the MTP.

Advice and help are provided by MTP therapy staff to assist teachers and other school staff in developing plans to meet the child's accessibility issues and other concerns related to function in the school.

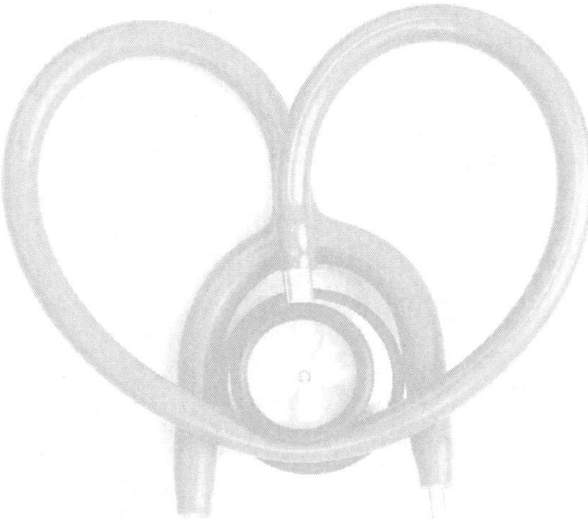

Miscellaneous Information

Normal Respiratory Rates

Ages	Breaths per minute
Infants	30–60
Toddlers	24–40
Preschoolers	22–34
School-age children	18–30
Adolescents	12–16

Greater than sixty breaths per minute always abnormal!

5 Point Respiratory Exam

1. Respiratory rate and rhythm
2. Skin color
3. Air entry
4. Work of breathing
5. Mental status

Signs of Respiratory Distress

- Increased work of breathing
- Increased respiratory rate
- Increased level of consciousness (agitated)
- Irregular breathing patterns
- Noisy breath sounds

Signs of Respiratory Failure

- Diminished breath sounds
- Altered muscle tone
- Cyanosis
- Decreased level of consciousness
- Decreased respiratory functions

Signs and Symptoms of Hypoxemia (Decreased Oxygen Level in Blood)

Dyspnea	Grunting
Confusion	Cyanosis
Restlessness	Retractions
Nasal flaring	Diaphoresis
Agitation	Tachypnea

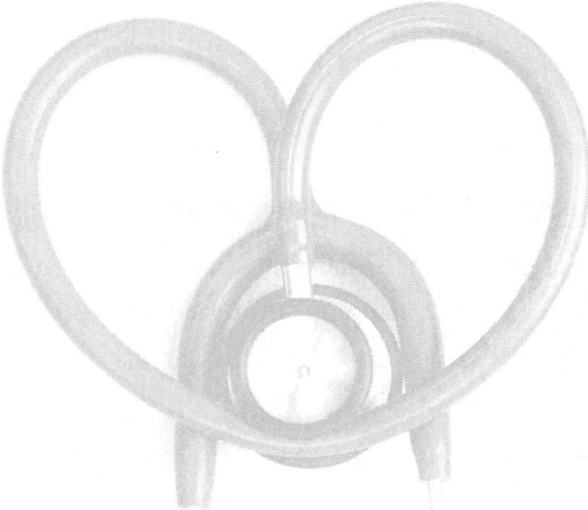

Who is Whom?

Audiologist: A medical professional who is specially trained to detect, diagnose, and treat individuals with impaired hearing.

Cardiac surgeon: One who specializes in performing surgery on the heart.

Cardiologist: A doctor who specializes in the heart and circulation of blood.

Gastroenterologist: One who specializes in the treatment of stomach and intestinal disorders.

Geneticist: One who studies birth defects and their causes.

Hematologist: One who specializes in diagnosis and treatment of blood problems.

Neonatal nurse practitioner (NNP): A registered nurse who has special training in the care of critically ill babies.

Neonatologist: Baby doctor (pediatrician) who has specialized training in the care of premature infants or critically ill newborns.

Neurologist: One who specializes in the diagnosis and treatment of brain and nervous system disorders.

Neurosurgeon: One who specializes in surgery on the brain and nervous system.

Occupational therapist (OT): One who treats problems involving the use of muscles, also may work with babies who have trouble eating.

Ophthalmologist: Doctor who specializes in eye problems.

Orthopedist: Doctor who specializes in bone problems.

Pediatric cardiologist: One who specializes in the diagnosis and treatment of heart problems in children.

Pediatric surgeon: One who specializes in performing surgery on newborns and children.

Physical therapist (PT): One who treats feeding problems and problems of the muscles.

Pulmonologist: One who specializes in diagnosis and treatment of certain lung conditions.

Resident: Doctor in training after medical school.

Respiratory therapist: Medical professional who is trained,

certified, and registered to set up, calibrate, monitor, and supervise the use of respiratory equipment.

Urologist: One who specializes in the diagnosis and treatment of urinary tract infections.

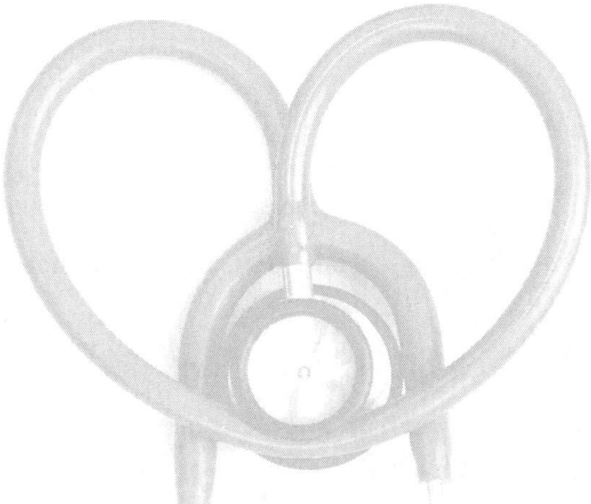

Definitions of Terms

Abdomen: The area between the chest and the hips in the front of the body.

Adjusted age (or corrected age): The age a premature baby would be if he or she had been born on his or her due date.

Adoption home study: The written document that explains the thorough background of a potential adoptive family, outlining their suitability as a potential adoptive home, as well as their current family and home dynamics.

Adoption placement papers: Paperwork indicating that the case plan for a child or children is permanency, specifying that the signing family intends to adopt said child/children.

Adoptive match: Assessment or match made by the DCFS Placement and Recruitment Unit (PRU) between a waiting family who has completed an adoption home study and a child or children who need an adoptive home.

Agitation: Excessive restlessness, increased mental and physical activity.

Allergy: hypersensitivity to normal environmental antigens.

Ambu bag: A piece of respiratory equipment. Used with a face mask and placed over baby's nose and mouth, or attached to ET tube or trach tube; it is squeezed to give the baby oxygen and inflate the lungs.

Anemia: A medical condition caused by abnormally low concentrations of red blood cells.

Angina: A choking, suffocation sense of pain.

Anomaly: Malformed body part.

Anorexia: Lack or loss of appetite for food.

Anoxia: Lack of oxygen.

Anuria: Absence of urine formation, manifested by no urine output.

Anus: The opening at the end of the large intestine. Stool leaves the body through this opening.

Apgar Score: A means of evaluation, on a scale of one to ten, how a newborn baby adjusts to the environment outside the uterus immediately after delivery.

Apnea: A breathing pause that lasts longer than fifteen to twenty seconds.

Areola: Dark area of the breast around the nipple.

Arteries: Large, thick-walled blood vessels that distribute oxygenated blood to the capillaries.

Asphyxia: A condition marked by a serious lack of sufficient oxygen and rising carbon dioxide levels that affects organ systems and could cause death or major problems if not rapidly treated and reversed.

Aspiration: Breathing fluid (formula, stomach contents, meconium [baby's first stool]) or objects into the lung.

Atelectasis: Condition in which lungs of a fetus remain unexpanded at birth. May be caused by obstruction by foreign bodies, mucus plugs, or excess secretions. In adults, collapse of a lung.

Bacteria: Germs that make you sick. Treated with antibiotics.

Bagging: Pumping air and/or oxygen into the baby's lungs by compression; a bag attached to a mask that covers the baby's nose and mouth.

Bililights (phototherapy): A mode of treatment for jaundice in which the baby is placed under special fluorescent lights that break down the structure of the bilirubin so it con be more easily transported to the liver and then excreted from the body.

Bilirubin: A yellowish red pigment found in small amounts in everyone's blood. Excess amounts sometimes produced in a baby's body cause him or her to develop jaundice.

BiPAP: A respiratory method that delivers a constant flow of air into the lungs. The flow is increased when the person breathes in. It is used for the treatment of apnea or chronic lung disease. BiPAP can be used at home with careful monitoring by parents and/or skilled nurses.

Birth defect: Any defect present in a baby at birth, irrespective of whether the defect is caused by a genetic factor or by prenatal events that are not genetic.

Blood gas analysis: A test to determine the oxygen, carbon dioxide, and acid content of the blood.

Bonding: A process by which a parent and child become emotionally attached.

Bradycardia: Slow heart rate, usually less than one hundred in a newborn or premature baby. A significant drop in the heart rate below the normal rate for that individual. Absolute bradycardia is generally a heartbeat below ninety beats per minute. However, for some babies, any significant drop below their normal rate may indicate relative bradycardia, which may be abnormal in certain situations and may have to be treated.

Brain bleed: Bleeding or hemorrhage into some part of the brain. See intraventricular hemorrhage.

Breech delivery: Baby born bottom, feet, or arms first.

Bronchopulmonary dysplasia (BPD): A chronic lung disease found in some babies who are on a respirator and/or extra oxygen for more than twenty-eight days. Also called chronic lung disease (CLD).

Candida Albicans (monilia or yeast infection): Infection that causes thrush and other yeast infections. Seen most often in baby's mouth or diaper area.

Cannula: A method of delivering oxygen. A thin flexible tube goes over the baby's face and head and is connected to an oxygen source. A flow meter regulates the amount of oxygen that is given to the baby through the two prongs that extend from the tube into the baby's nostrils.

Carbon dioxide: Gas breathed out when the baby exhales.

Cardiac output: Amount of blood ejected by the heart in one minute.

Cardiopulmonary resuscitation (CPR): Method to revive a person whose heartbeat and breathing have stopped or slowed abnormally.

Case plan: The requirements set by the court that must be fulfilled by the birth family in order to reunify with a child or children.

Catheter: A narrow, flexible tube used to give fluids to the body or to drain fluids from the body.

Cerebrospinal fluid (CSF): Fluid made and stored in the ventricles of the brain; same as spinal fluid.

Chest physiotherapy (CPT): Clapping on the baby's chest with a hand or using a cup to loosen mucus in the lungs.

Circumcision: Removal of the foreskin from the penis.

Clinodactyly: Permanent deviation or deflection of one or more fingers.

Clubbing: Proliferation of soft tissue about the terminal phalanges of fingers or toes without bone change.

Colic: Daily period of crying for three hours or more during which the infant is virtually inconsolable.

Colostomy: A surgically created opening in the abdominal wall that allows the colon (the lower section of the large intestine) to empty directly into a waste bag outside the body.

Colostrum: The yellowish fluid secreted from the breasts before the mother's milk comes in. It is several times higher in protein than the later milk.

Complete blood count (CBC): Blood test that looks at the types and number of cells in the blood.

Computerized axial tomography (CAT scan or CT scan): Computerized X-ray that takes special pictures of the baby's brain.

Concurrent planning: The long-term case plan for a child that includes both the possibility of reunifying with the birth family and the possibility of being adopted by the foster family.

Congenital abnormality: Birth defect, malformation, or abnormality present at birth.

Congenital heart disease (CHD): Any heart disease that a baby is born with.

Congestive heart failure (CHF): Heart is not able to pump blood well because of malformed heart, illness, or infection.

Constriction: A narrowing or compression of a part. Atelectasis in the newborn also causes grunting because of the work required for the baby to fill the lungs.

Continuous positive airway pressure (CPAP): A respiratory method that forces a constant flow of air into the lungs through a narrow tube placed in one or both nostrils. Also called positive end expiratory pressure (PEEP).

Corrected age: length of pregnancy (gestational age) plus the baby's calendar age.

County counsel: Legal counsel representing the Department of Children and Family Services.

Court order: A legal order given by the dependency court pertaining to the child or children's case that must be followed as directed by the issuing judge.

Cryptorchid: A person with undescended testes.

Cyanosis: A term used to describe blueness of the skin, generally caused by lack of oxygen.

Cytomegalovirus (CMV): A virus the baby can get before he is born that causes birth defects and illness. He can also get it after birth, and it can cause illness.

Dehydration: Deficiency in body fluid from decreased intake, output greater than intake, or loss of fluids by vomiting, diarrhea, or diaphoresis.

Dependency court: The legal court system handling all dependency court cases. This is not civil or criminal court.

Detention: The action of removing a child from their current caretaker. Children can be detained if there is a reasonable suspicion that a child has been abused, abandoned, neglected, or when it is assessed that a child is at imminent risk of harm should he or she remain in the care, custody, or control of their caretaker.

Detention hearing (seventy-two-hour hearing): The first

court hearing held following a detention. At this hearing, the caretaker will be told why their child or children were detained and what they must do to reunify. Further, a determination is made as to whether or not there is an appropriate relative who can care for the child and visitation rights are established.

Developmental assessment: Measurement of physical, cognitive, psychosocial, and psychosexual parameters compared to norms for one's chronologic age.

Developmental problems: These kinds of problems include a lag in motor coordination skills (such as lifting the head up, rolling over, sitting, standing, or walking), hearing or vision impairment, behavioral problems such as extreme irritability or inconsolability, and learning disabilities.

Diaphoresis: Perspiration, especially profuse perspiration.

Diaphragm: The big muscle below the lungs that controls breathing.

Diuretic: Drug used to get rid of extra body water.

Doppler: Special blood pressure machine.

Down syndrome: Chromosome abnormality (Trisomy 21) where the baby has varying physical problems and varying degrees of mental retardation.

Dyspnea: Labored breathing.

Early intervention program: A method of physical therapy that may help a child to use his or her muscles fully and reach maximum motor potential.

Echocardiogram: An ultrasonograhic method of recording a picture of the heart as it is produced by the echo of sound waves. This can be used to evaluate both the structure and function of the heart.

Edema: Swelling or puffiness.

Electrocardiogram (EKG): a record of the electrical activity of the heart.

Electroencephalogram (EEG): A method of recording and analyzing the electrical activity of the brain.

Electrolytes: Chemicals in the body that make it function well; can be checked by drawing blood for lab work.

Emergency response worker (ER worker): an employee that responds to the initial allegation of abuse or neglect by going to the home and determining if the child is in imminent risk of harm. The ER worker is the worker that makes the critical decision whether or not a child should be detained.

Encephalitis: Encephalitis refers to inflammation of the tissues of the brain resulting from invasion from a toxic or infectious agent, usually a virus and is almost always associated with alteration of mental status.

Encrustation: Hard, crusty, dried mucus.

Endogenous: Produced within or caused by factors within the organism.

Endotracheal tube (ET tube): small plastic tube placed in the nose or throat and connected to a ventilator or breathing machine. The tube is in the baby's breathing passage (trachea) and delivers oxygen and pressure to the lungs.

Enterocolitis: Infection of the small and large intestines.

Epithelium: Cellular substance of skin and mucous membrane.

Erythropoietin: A glycoprotein hormone secreted by the kidney in the adult and by the liver in the fetus that acts on stem cells of the bone marrow to stimulate red blood cell production.

Esophagus: The tube that connects the stomach to the throat; about nine inches long.

Evoked potential testing (auditory brain stem response studies or brain stem auditory evoked response studies): a neurologic diagnostic procedure that determines a baby's potential for hearing.

Exchange transfusion: removing most of the baby's blood in small amounts and replacing it with fresh blood in small amounts; most often used for a very high bilirubin level.

Excoriation: Rubbing away of part of the skin by disease or injury.

Exhale: To breathe out.

Expiration: Breathe out.

Extra corporeal membrane oxygenation (ECMO): Process used to circulate a baby's blood in a special machine while his lungs rest. It is a type of heart pump like those used on adults having heart surgery. Babies may stay on the pump for more than a week. They would also be on a breathing machine.

Extubation: Take out the endotracheal (breathing) tube (ET tube).

Fellow: A licensed doctor who is completing a two- to

three-year training period before taking an exam to become a certified specialist.

Finalization: A court preceding that makes an adoption legal and binding.

Flatus: Stomach or intestinal gas.

Fontannel: Space covered by membranous tissue at the juncture of cranial sutures.

Fraternal twins: Twins formed from two fertilized eggs. They do not look alike. There can be a boy and a girl or two girls or two boys.

Full term: Baby born between the thirty-eighth and forty-second week of pregnancy or gestation.

Ganglion cells: A type of nerve cell involved in moving stool through the large intestine. A person with Hirschsprung's disease is missing these cells from part of the large intestine.

Gastrostomy: Surgical hole on the tummy into the stomach. A tube is placed in the stomach to feed babies unable to eat by mouth.

Gavage feeding: Feeding by a tube placed in the baby's nose or mouth into the stomach.

Gestational age: The age of the fetus and newborn, which is calculated by counting the weeks from the mother's last menstrual period before conception. Full-term is forty weeks gestation.

Glottis: The space between the vocal cords.

Glucose: A type of simple sugar that supplies the body with energy.

Gram (gm, G, GM): Weight in metric system. One ounce equals twenty-eight grams.

Gram-negative organisms: Any number of bacteria that may find their way into the baby's respiratory system or blood through a respirator tube or during the process of delivery.

Gross motor skills: Skills requiring the use of large muscle groups, such as head control, sitting, standing, and walking.

Group B strep infection: Type of bacterial infection that a baby can get from the mother during the birthing process.

Grunting: Abnormal, short, loud breaks in breathing out. They often happen with severe chest pain. The grunt is made as the glottis briefly stops the flow of air, halting the movement of the lungs and their surrounding structures.

Head circumference: Measurement of the largest diameter of the head.

Heat shield: A device that intensifies the heat from the artificial heat source of the radiant warmer or incubator.

Heel stick: Method to prick heel (finger stick is used also) to get blood for lab tests.

Hemarthrosis: Bleeding into a joint.

Hematocrit (hct or crit): Percent of red blood cells in the blood. Your baby may receive a transfusion based on the hemocrit.

Hematuria: Blood in the urine.

Hematologist: A doctor who specializes in blood problems.

High-risk baby: Baby at risk for developmental problems. Includes babies with intracranial hemorrhages, birth weight less than 1,200 grams, long-term breathing machine (ventilators), less than thirty weeks gestation, small for gestational age babies, congenital infections, meningitis, birth defects, etc.

Hives: Skin rash characterized by large welts.

House officer: Doctor who is finishing his training; a resident or fellow.

House staff: Doctors who are finishing their training; residents and fellows.

Hyaline membrane disease (HMD): Also called respiratory distress syndrome (RDS) a breathing problem of premature infants caused by lack of a fluid called surfactant that keeps small air sacs in the lungs open.

Hydrocephalus: An abnormal accumulation of spinal fluid in the ventricles of the brain, which is characterized by an abnormal increase in head size and a progressive loss of brain tissue.

Hyperbilirubinemia: High bilirubin level (yellow jaundice); common in newborns. Some babies are placed under a special light (bili light) or blanket that helps the body breakdown the bilirubin. The baby gets rid of the bilirubin in his stools.

Hyperosmolarity: Abnormally increased osmolar concentration.

Hypertension: High blood pressure.

Hypertrophy: The enlargement of a tissue or organ owing to an increase in the size of its constituent cells.

Hyponatremia: Deficiency of sodium in the blood; salt depletion.

Hypotonia: Deficient muscle tone.

Hypovolemia: Abnormally decreased volume of circulation fluid in the body.

Hypoxia: A lack of sufficient oxygen.

Identical twins: Twins that occur from the division of a single fertilized egg. They are the same sex and look alike.

Ileostomy: A surgical procedure that creates a diversion of the intestine for the drainage of stool into a bag. This procedure is sometimes used to treat problems such as intestinal obstruction or necrotizing enterocolitis.

Immunization: Medicines given to protect the child against harmful childhood diseases; given by mouth or by shot.

Inborn: Baby born in the same hospital with a neonatal intensive care unit.

Infusion pump: A device attached to an intravenous line that carefully regulates, in precisely measured amounts, the fluids going into a baby's bloodstream.

Inflammation: Changes, such as redness, swelling, pain, and heat, that occur in living tissues when they are invaded by germs.

Inguinal hernia: Lump under the skin in the groin or scrotum caused by the intestines pushing through a weak place in the belly wall; a common preemie problem. May be fixed by surgery before the baby leaves the hospital.

Inhale: To breathe in.

Inherent: Intrinsic, innate.

Inspiration: Breathe in.

Intermittent mandatory ventilation: A respiratory device in which a tube is threaded through the baby's nose or mouth, down the back of the throat, and into the trachea. IMV is most often used in a harmonious pattern with the baby's own breathing rate in order to adequately oxygenate and ventilate the child.

Intracranial hemorrhage (ICH): Bleeding in or around the brain.

Intravenous (IV): Tube or needle placed in the vein to give fluids, medications, or blood.

Intraventricular hemorrhage (intracranial hemorrhage or brain bleed): A medical condition that results from abnormal bleeding on the surface of the brain, in the substance of the brain, or in the brain's central chambers that are continuous with the canal of the spinal cord.

Intubation: The insertion of a tube into the trachea (windpipe) through the nose or mouth to allow air to reach the lungs.

In utero: Inside the womb or uterus.

Isolette: An incubator (plastic box) the baby is placed in to keep him warm while he grows and gets well.

Jaundice (hyperbilirubinemia): a condition that occurs when there is an overabundance of bilirubin in the body.

Jet ventilator: Special breathing machine that uses fast rates to breathe for babies who have special lung problems.

Kilogram: Unit of weight in the metric system. 1kg = 2.2 pounds; 1kg = 1,000 grams.

Lactation: Making milk in the breast.

Lactation consultant: An experienced professional who can give practical tips and encouragement about the process of breastfeeding.

Lactose: Sugar in breast milk or formula.

Lanugo: Fine hair that covers the body of a fetus and some premature babies.

Legal guardianship: The long-term placement plan for children who cannot be reunified with their birth family but either cannot or are not willing to be adopted.

Let-down reflex: flow of milk into the nipple.

Liquid ventilation: A respiratory technique that pumps lung fluids into the lungs through an endotracheal tube and replaces the air-lung function with a fluid-lung function to re-create the in utero environment and keep the air sacs expanded.

Low birth weight infant (LBW): Baby who weighs less than five pounds at birth; can be premature or full-term.

Lumbar puncture (LP, spinal tap): Procedure where a hollow needle is inserted between the bones in the back to withdraw spinal fluid.

Lumen: Inside part of the tube where the air goes in and out.

Meconium: Baby's first bowel movement; green-black color and sticky. Sometimes baby has a stool while in the uterus before birth.

Meconium aspiration: Breathing the meconium and amniotic fluid into the lungs.

MediCal: The insurance coverage for all medical, dental, and psychological services needed by foster and adoptive children.

Meningitis: Infection of the lining of the brain and spinal cord.

Meningocele: Birth defect where the tissue lining the brain and spinal cord come out through an opening in the skull or spinal column.

Metabolism: The sum of the physical and chemical processes by which living organized substance is built up and maintained and by which large molecules are broken down into smaller molecules to make energy available to the organism.

Milliliter (ml): Unit of volume. 5 ml = 1 teaspoon; 30 ml = 1 ounce.

Monilia: Yeast infection found in the baby's mouth or diaper area.

Monitor: A machine that records information such as heartbeat, body temperature, respiratory rate, and blood pressure.

Monitored visitation: Court-ordered visitation that takes place between a child and his/her family members or close family friends. Approved persons monitor these visits in order to ensure the safety of the child or children.

Mucus: Sticky material made in the nose and throat.

Murmur: Sound made by blood flowing through the heart.

Myopia: Nearsightedness.

Nasogastric tube: A narrow, flexible tube that is inserted through the nostril, down the esophagus, and into the stomach. It is used to deliver nourishment or to remove air or fluid from the stomach.

Navel: Belly button; umbilicus.

Nebulizer treatment: A method of delivering medication at home through a device that transforms medicine into droplet form for inhalation. Used for a variety of lung problems.

Necrosis: Death of a part of the body due to absence of blood supply.

Necrotizing enterocolitis (NEC): an infection of the intestines that sometimes results in part of the intestines dying. The dying part is removed by surgery.

Neonate: Baby during the first month of life.

Neonatal period: The first twenty-eight days of life.

Neonatal nurse practitioner (NNP): A registered nurse who has special training in the care of critically ill babies. A NNP may give medical care, discharge teaching, and other types of care under the supervision of a doctor; performs special procedures.

Neonatologist: Baby doctor (pediatrician) who has specialized training in the care of premature infants or critically ill newborns.

Nephritis: Inflammation of the kidneys.

Nephrons: The structural and functional unit of the kidney; numbering about a million in the renal parenchyma, each being capable of forming urine.

Nerve cells: Nerves are long fibers that carry messages from the body to the brain and back again, like telephone lines. The messages often tell a body part what to do. Nerve cells are part of nerves. In the intestine, the nerve cells tell muscles how to push the stool along.

Neurogenci: A term used to indicate anything that originates from within the nervous energy.

Neurologist: A doctor who specializes in problems of the brain and nervous system.

Nippling: Sucking on a bottle filled with formula or breast milk.

Nocturia: Bedwetting; frequent urination at night.

Nosocomial infections: Bacterial or other types of infections acquired directly from the hospital environment through any point where there is a breakdown in the skin's surface, such as IV or catheter sites, respiratory and feeding tubes, and any surgical incisions. Staphylococcus epidermidis and Staphylococcus aureus infections are examples of this kind of infection.

Nystagmus: Involuntary, rapid, jerky movement of the eye.

Oligohydramnios: Deficiency in the amount of amniotic fluid.

Oliguria: Decreased urine formation manifested by low urine output.

Orogastric tube: A narrow, flexible tube that is threaded through the mouth, down the esophagus, and into the stomach. It is used to deliver nourishment or to remove air or fluid from the stomach.

Osmolality: The concentration of a solution in terms of osmoles of solutes per kilogram of solvent.

Osteoporosis: A disorder that causes a gradual decrease in both the amount and strength of bone tissue.

Ostomy: Surgery to connect part of the intestine to a hole in the abdomen.

Ototoxic antibiotics: Drugs used to fight infections. They have the potential to cause hearing problems.

Outborn: Baby transported from another hospital for care after his birth.

Parenteral nutrition (hyperalimentation): A solution fed directly into the baby's bloodstream that gives him or her necessary nutrients such as carbohydrates, electrolytes, protein, minerals, vitamins, and fat.

Patent ductus arteriosus (PDA): Small vessel outside of the heart that sometimes fails to close after birth. Sometimes it is closed with medicine or by surgery. Sometimes it causes the baby to have breathing and heart problems.

PEEP: Positive end expiratory pressure.

Perforated bowel: A hole in the intestine.

Perinatal period: The time immediately before, during, or after birth.

Periodic breathing: A type of breathing pattern. The baby will stop breathing for a few seconds; then breathes quickly.

Peristalsis: The normal movements of the intestines that move the food along the digestive tract.

Persistent fetal circulation (PFC) or Persistent pulmonary hypertension of the newborn (PPHN): At birth, the circulation and breathing changes. In PPHN, the baby's blood flow does not change and continues to bypass the lungs. When this happens, the body and brain do not get enough oxygen.

Petechia: A minute red spot due to escape of a small amount of blood.

Phototherapy: Treatment of yellow jaundice or high bilirubin by placing the baby under bright light (bililight) or on a blanket (bili blanket).

Placenta abruptio: Placenta pulls away from the wall of the uterus (womb). There is often bleeding. A caesarean delivery is often needed.

Placenta previa: Placenta is located in an abnormal place (over the opening of the womb). Bleeding during the pregnancy can occur. Caesarean (C-section) delivery is often needed.

Pneumogram (Sleep Study): Twelve or twenty-four-hour recording of the baby's breathing and heart rate patterns to see if there are unusual patterns during sleep or feeding.

Postpartum: Time lasting six weeks after mom delivers a baby.

Postural drainage: Method of positioning a baby so mucus can drain from the lungs.

Premature baby (Preterm Baby): Baby born before the end of the thirty-seventh week of pregnancy.

Premature rupture of the membranes (PROM): The bag of water (amniotic fluid) the baby floats in leaks or breaks before labor.

Prenatal: Before birth.

Primary nurse: Nurse who is responsible for providing care and coordinating care of a specific baby for entire time baby is in the unit.

Prostaglandins: Naturally occurring substances in the body that affect the cardiovascular system by altering the blood flow to a variety of organs. Different classifications of prostaglandins may selectively increase or inhibit the blood flow to a particular organ.

Pruritus: Itching.

Pseudomonas: A genus of gram-negative, strictly anaerobic bacteria that causes various human diseases.

Pulse oximeter: Machine that reads the oxygen saturation of blood. The pulse oximeter is taped to baby's hand, finger, or toe.

Radiant warmer: An open bed with a heat source that allows immediate access to newborn and sick preemies while maintaining a warm air temperature.

Rectum: The last section of the large intestine.

Residual: Formula still in the stomach before the next feeding.

Respirator: Machine used to breath for the baby. Also called a ventilator.

Respite care: Supervision of children, provided by an alternate provider, while the primary foster parent(s) are out of town or unable to care for the child or children.

Retina: The back of the eye.

Retinopathy of prematurity (ROP): An eye disease in babies. Many things, including oxygen, ventilators, and prematurity, may cause it. The mild form may heal on its own, but severe ROP may lead to the retina becoming detached (loose) and blindness.

Retractions: The act of drawing back, such as the skin drawing back between the ribs in respiratory distress.

Reunification: The act of returning the care, custody, and control of a child to his or her birth family, a relative, or previous caretaker.

Reunification services: Services funded and facilitated by the county, as per the court-ordered case plan, provided with the goal of rehabilitating and preparing the birth family to reunify with their child or children.

Rubella: Virus that causes German measles.

Scoliosis: Lateral curvature of vertebral column.

Sedation: Allaying irritability and excitement.

Seizure: Abnormal electrical activity in the brain that causes unusual muscle twitches.

Sepsis: A medical condition in which there is bacteria in the bloodstream. The bacteria travel in the blood to many parts of the body and cause notable changes in the health condition.

Septic shock: A body infection that causes a drop in the stability of the vital signs due to a decrease in heart functioning.

Shunt (VP): Tube that drains spinal fluid from a ventricle in the brain to the belly.

Spinal tap (lumbar puncture): A diagnostic procedure in which a short, narrow needle is inserted between two lumbar vertebrae into the area where there is spinal fluid. The spinal fluid is withdrawn for analysis.

Status asthmaticus: Acute asthma exacerbation in which there's unrelenting, severe respiratory distress and bronchospasm.

Steatorrhea: More than normal amounts of fat in the feces resulting in foamy, light-colored, bulky, foul-smelling, greasy stools.

Stenosis: Constricted; decrease in diameter.

Stipend: Money paid to the foster parent(s) as a reimbursement for expenses incurred while caring for the foster child or children.

Stoma: A hole on the outside of the body made by surgery. Stool leaves the body through the hole instead of through the anus.

Strabismus: Eyes that cross or turn outward due to muscle weakness.

Subarachnoid hemorrhage: Bleeding in the area around the outside of the brain.

Submicroscopic: Too small to be visible with the microscope.

Sudden infant death syndrome (SIDS): Sudden death of a previously healthy infant in which a postmortem examination fails to confirm the cause of death.

Surfactant: Phospholipid that lines the alveoli, preventing them from collapsing during exhalation.

Tachycardia: Rapid heart rate (above 160 beats per minute in a newborn or premature).

Tachypnea: Unusually fast rate of breathing.

Technical assistant (TA): A county employee that contacts foster family agencies and county licensed homes when looking for an appropriate foster care placement.

Term baby: Baby born between the thirty-eighth and forty-second week of pregnancy (gestation).

Termination: The end of foster care placement.

Termination of parental rights (TPR): A court order severing parental rights from the biological parents based on the parents' failure to comply with the case plan.

Thrush: Fungal (yeast) infection of the mouth. Baby has white patches on the tongue and insides of the mouth.

TORCH titers: Test for viral infections toxoplasmosis, rubella, cytomegalovirus, and herpes.

Trachea: Windpipe or breathing tube.

Tracheotomy: Surgical opening made through the skin

and into the breathing tube (trachea) so air can get to the lungs when there is a blockage. Also done to babies requiring long-term ventilation management.

Transfer: The movement of a child from one foster home to another. Transfers are often done to accommodate placing sibling sets together, to move children closer to their birth families, and/or to be placed into a permanent adoptive home.

Transfusion: A treatment for anemia in which red blood cells are added directly to the baby's total circulating blood supply through an IV or a catheter.

Ultrasound: Method of taking pictures inside the body using sound waves.

Umbilical hernia: A pushing out of the navel or belly button caused by the intestines pushing through a weak place in the belly wall; usually goes away by the age of two; fixed by surgery after two to three years of age if still present.

Umbilicus: Belly button; navel.

Unmonitored visitation: Court-ordered visitation that takes place between a child and his or her family members or close family friends whom the court does not deem necessary to be monitored for the safety of the child or children.

Ureter: The tube that carries the urine from the bladder to the outside.

Ureterostomy: A creation of a new outlet for a ureter.

Urticaria: Hives.

Ventilator: Machine used to breathe for the baby; also called a respirator.

Ventricle: Chamber in the heart; also the name of a sack in the brain where spinal fluid is made and stored.

Wheeze: Whistling, humming, raspy sound made during breathing.

Yeast infection (Candida albicans, monilia, thrush): Fungus that causes an infection; common after antibiotic therapy. Seen most often in the mouth and diaper area. Treated with mycostatin oral suspension and mycostatin cream.

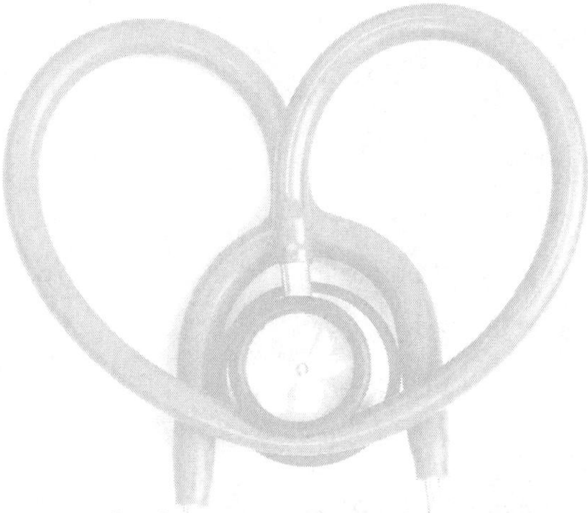

Abbreviations

A & B: apnea and bradycardia

ABG: arterial blood gas

ac: before meals

ADLs: activities of daily living

ad lib: freely as desired

AIDS: acquired immunodeficiency syndrome

Algo: hearing screens

ALL: acute lymphocytic leukemia

AMA: against medical advice

ASA: acetylsalicylic acid

BE: barium enema

bid: Dose twice a day or every twelve hours

Bili: Bilirubin

BP: blood pressure

BPD: bronchopulmonary dysplasia

BRP: bathroom privileges

BUN: blood urea nitrogen

cap: capsule

CBC: complete blood count

cc or ml: metric measures of liquid; 30cc (or ml) is 1 ounce; 5 cc is approximately 1 teaspoon

CDC: Centers for Disease Control and Prevention

CHF: congestive heart failure

CNS: central nervous system (brain and spinal cord) or clinical nurse specialist

c/o: complains of

CO: carbon monoxide

CPAP: continuous positive airway pressure (air or oxygen delivered under a small amount of pressure)

CPR: cardiopulmonary resuscitation

CPT or Chest PT: chest physiotherapy (vibrating or tapping on the chest)

CT: computed tomography

DPT: diphtheria, pertussis, tetanus; one of the baby shots or immunizations

DNR: do not resuscitate

Dx: diagnosis

ET: Endotracheal (refers to a tube placed through the mouth or nose to the wind pipe)

EEG: electroencephalogram; tracing of the electrical impulses of the brain

elix: elixir

EKG: electrocardiogram; tracing of the electrical impulses of the heart

ER: emergency room

ETOH: ethyl alcohol

FDA: Food and Drug Administration

FUO: fever of unknown origin

Fx: Fracture

GI: gastrointestinal

Gms or grams: Metric weight; 450 grams equals 1 pound; 1 kilogram (Kg) equals 1,000 grams

gr: grain

gt, gtt: drop, drops

GTT: glucose tolerance test

HCT: hematocrit

Hgb: hemoglobin

HMD: hyaline membrane disease (another name for respiratory distress syndrome)

HI-FI: high-frequency ventilator

HIV: human immunodeficiency virus

hr: hour

HR: heart rate

H&P: history and physical examination

hs: at bedtime

HSV: herpes simplex virus

ID: infectious disease or identification

IDM: infant of a diabetic mother

IDDM: insulin-dependent diabetes mellitus

IEP: individualized educational plan

IM: intramuscular

IMV: intermittent mandatory ventilation; number of breaths per minute by the ventilator

I & O: intake and output

IV: intravenous (by vein)

IVH: intraventricular hemorrhage

kg: kilogram

KVO: keep vein open

lb: pound

L: liter

LOC: level of consciousness

LP: lumbar puncture (getting sample of spinal fluid using a needle)

LPN: licensed practical nurse

LVN: licensed vocational nurse

mcg: microgram

mg: milligram

MI: myocardial infarction

mL: milliliter

MS: multiple sclerosis

MTP: medical therapy program

MTU: medical therapy unit

NDST: neuro development screening test

NEC: necrotizing enterocolitis

NG: nasal gastric (tube going from nose to stomach)

NICU: neonatal intensive care unit

NPO: nothing by mouth

NSAID: nonsteroidal anti-inflammatory drug

O^2: oxygen

O.D.: right eye

OG: oral gastric (tube going from mouth to stomach)

O.S.: left eye

OTC: over-the-counter

O.U.: both eyes

OT: occupational therapist

PDA: patent ductus arteriosus

PERRLA: pupils equal, round and reactive to light and accommodation

pH: hydrogen ion concentration

PIC or PCVL: a tiny catheter or tube placed into a vein to give fluids or nutrition

PICC: tiny catheter inserted into vein to give fluids and nutrition

P.O.: Given by mouth.

PT: physical therapist

PRN: as often as necessary; when required

PVCs: premature ventricular contractions

q: each, every

qid: dose four times per day. If a medication is ordered Q 6 hours, it is not the same as QID. QID is during normal waking hours.

Q 6 hours: around the clock

Q day: dose once a day

Qhs: every bedtime

RDS: respiratory distress syndrome

ROM: range of motion

RN: registered nurse

ROP: retinopathy of prematurity

RSV: respiratory syncytial virus

RRT: registered respiratory therapist

Rx: take; treatment

SIDS: sudden infant death syndrome

SIMV: synchronized intermittent mandatory ventilation (machine breaths timed to baby's)

Stat: immediately

SQ: subcutaneous

TB: tuberculosis

tid: three times a day

TLC: tender loving care

TPN or TNA: total parenteral nutrition (nutrition by vein)

TPR: temperature, pulse, and respiration

TTNB: transient tachypnea of the newborn

UAC: umbilical artery catheter; see equipment

URI: upper respiratory infection; a cold; infection above the lungs

UTI: urinary tract (kidney or bladder) infection

UVC: umbilical venous catheter; see equipment

VRE: vancomycin-resistant enterococcus

VS: vital signs (temperature, pulse, respiration, blood pressure)

WBC: white blood cell, white blood count

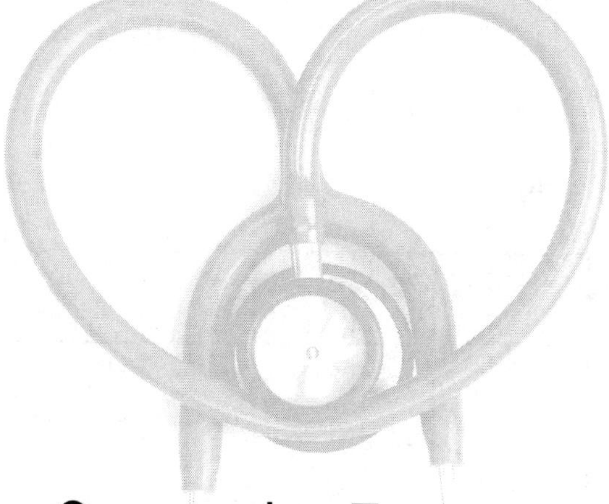

Sample Forms and Checklists

Name: Child's Name Date of Birth: 01/01/08

Medication name	Medical condition	Start date	End date	Dosage	Results	Side effects
Reglan	GI reflux		current	0.5ml	Decrease GI reflux	Sedation, fatigue, restlessness, headache
Pepcid	GI reflux		current	1.6ml BID	Decrease GI reflux	Nausea, constipation, Increase appetite
Albuterol	Lung disease		current	1 vial every 4 hours PRN	Decrease wheezing	Restlessness, Nervousness
Tylenol	Pain or increase temperature		current	0.4ml every 4 hours PRN	Decrease temp, Decrease pain	Rare side effects, rash

INDIVIDUALIZED HEALTH CARE PLAN

Name: Child's name Updated: 01/01/01

Problem #1 Alteration in feeding mode and behaviors R/T G-tube placement secondary to failure to thrive, and severe prematurity.

Goal/objective:

1. Maintain tube placement.
2. Maintain calorie intake via G-tube to support nutrition.
3. Increase feedings to a degree that will support total nutritional needs for optimum growth and development.

Interventions:

1. Caregivers will follow orders prescribed by MD for feeding program.
2. Document results of feedings to assess need to change or readiness to learn new skills.
3. Follow outlined program consistently to promote maximum effectiveness and to see need for any alterations in program plan.

Evaluation:

INDIVIDUALIZED HEALTH CARE PLAN

Problem #2 Potential for alteration of skin integrity R/T stoma secondary to G-tube placement.

Goal/objective: G-tube site will be free of any S/S of infection AEB:

1. No drainage
2. No redness > 1/8 inch.
3. No foul odor.
4. Intact skin around stoma site.

Interventions:

1. Daily care of stoma, wash with warm water and mild soap at bath time.
2. Assess and document any increasing redness, drainage, or foul odor.
3. Observe for any S/S of systemic infection AEB: increased temperature or increasing irritability.

Evaluation: This area is where you would explain how the child is currently doing and how the interventions are affecting the goals and progress of the child. Usually the care plan is written by the registered nurse following the child and evaluation is done approximately every six months.

INDIVIDUALIZED HEALTH CARE PLAN

Problem #3 Alternation in growth and development R/T environmental/stimulation deficiencies secondary to medically fragile condition and prenatal drug exposure.

Goal/objective: (child's name) will reach his maximum potential in mental and physical development AEB:

1. Satisfactory/consistent growth, weight gain, and wellness.
2. (Child's name) will experience constructive parenting such as holding, rocking, playing, etc.
3. (Child's name) will demonstrate increased self-care skills.

Interventions:

1. Staff will monitor nutritional status and tolerance of program.
2. Monitor weight monthly.
3. Administer prescribed formula.
4. Provide stimulation and develop self-care skills.
5. Staff and foster family will provide sensory stimulation such as holding, talking, songs, and playing.

Evaluation:

INDIVIDUALIZED HEALTH CARE PLAN

Problem #4 High risk for injury R/T altered level of consciousness secondary to increased ICP and/or shunt malfunction

Goal/objectives: (Child's name) will have no sign of further injury AEB maintaining neurologic function.

Interventions:

1. Assess (child's name) neurologic status q 8 hours for the following:
    A. altered level of consciousness
    B. high-pitched cry
    C. irritability when awake
    D. lethargy
2. Assess for S/S of shunt infection such as:
    A. swelling along shunt tract
    B. increased temperature
    C. projectile vomiting
3. Assess vital signs every 8 hours noting irregularities in respiration and heart rate.

Evaluation:

Inventory list

Shoes_____

Socks_____

One piece outfits (shorts)_____

One piece outfits (long)_______

Pants_____

Shirts_____ Sleepers_______

PJ's______ Sweat outfits_______

T-shirts_____

Equipment_______

____

____

____

____

____

____

Toys__________

____

____

____

Name:							
	Date of each seizure:						
	Time of onset:						
	Total Time Involved:						
Place checks in appropriate columns to right:							
OBSERVATION BEFORE SEIZURE							
	cries out						
	Other						
OBSERVATION DURING SEIZURE							
Extremities:	Upper and lower						
Arms	Right						
	Left						
Legs	Right						
	Left						
	straight						
	Bent						
	Stiff						

	Limp						
Verbal sounds:	before						
	During						
Face twitching:							
Mouth:	Open						
	closed						
	grimacing						
Drooling:							
Vomited:							
Eye movement:	staring						
	Open						
	closed						
	fluttering						
	Rolled back						
Head:	Turned right						
	Turned left						
	Turned down						
	hyperextended back						
	nodding						
Body-trunk:	Rigid						
	Limp						
	Sitting						
	Laying						
	trembling						

	jerking						
	standing						
Skin color:	Pale						
	Gray						
	Blue						
	red (flushed)						
Breathing:	difficulty during						
	difficulty after						
	15 seconds						
	1 minute						
	longer (chart length)						
	Oxygen applied						
Incontinent:	bladder						
	bowel						
OBSERVATION AFTER SEIZURE	drowsy						
	confused						
	slept (chart length)						
Other:	Injury						
doctor notified							

911 notified if longer then 5 minutes							
Additional comments or observations as follows:							
Signature:							

Training Checklist for Bronchopulmonary Dysplasia

____ Reviewed the pathophysiology of bronchopulmonary dysplasia and state the S/S of respiratory distress.

____ State the S/S of apnea and bradycardia of prematurely.

____ Reviewed with demonstration all medications, dosage, frequency and possible side effects.

____ Instructed and return demonstration on the use of apnea monitor, how to respond to an alarm, assess the situation, and possible interventions.

____ Instructed with return demonstration of mixing of proper formula,

frequency, and maintenance. Discussed feeding goals, feedingschedule, and techniques.

____ Instructed on S/S of increased oxygen requirements, and respiratory distress. Interventions discussed such as oxygen via mask and/ornasal cannula.

____ Instructed with return demonstration oxygen delivery system, how to control flow, read dials, and order oxygen as needed.

Signature/titleofpersontrained:______________________
Date: ______

Signature/title of trainer:___________________________
Date: _______

1 hour

Training Checklist for Cardiac Disease

____ Reviewed all medications, dosage, frequency and possible side effects.

____ Instructed on clinical manifestations and pathophysiology of heart and lung condition.

____ Instructed on S/S of increased oxygen requirements, and respiratory distress. Interventions discussed such as oxygen via mask or nasal cannula, calming Coral and/or calling 911.

____ Instructed with return demonstration of mixing of proper formula, frequently, and maintenance. Discussed feeding goals, feeding schedule and techniques.

____ Instructed with return demonstration on GT site cleaning, and S/S of site infection.

____ Instructed with return demonstration on GT feedings, frequency, medication administration and adverse effects of GT feedings.

Signature/title of person trained: ____________________ Date: ________

Signature/title of trainer: __________________________ Date: ________

1 hour

Child's Name: ____________________________

Visitors Sign In Sheet

Date: _____ Time In: ________

Name/Relationship: __________________________

Time Out: ______ Signature: __________________

Date: _____ Time In: ________

Name/Relationship: __________________________

Time Out: ______ Signature: __________________

Date: _____ Time In: ________

Name/Relationship: __________________________

Time Out: ______ Signature: __________________

Date: _____ Time In: ________

Name/Relationship: __________________________

Time Out: ______ Signature: __________________

Date: _____ Time In: ________

Name/Relationship: __________________________

Time Out: ______ Signature: __________________

Date: _____ Time In: ________

Name/Relationship: __________________________

Time Out: ______ Signature: __________________

Date: _____ Time In: ________

Name/Relationship: __________________________

Time Out: ______ Signature: ________________

Date: _____ Time In: ________

Name/Relationship: __________________________

Time Out: ______ Signature: ________________

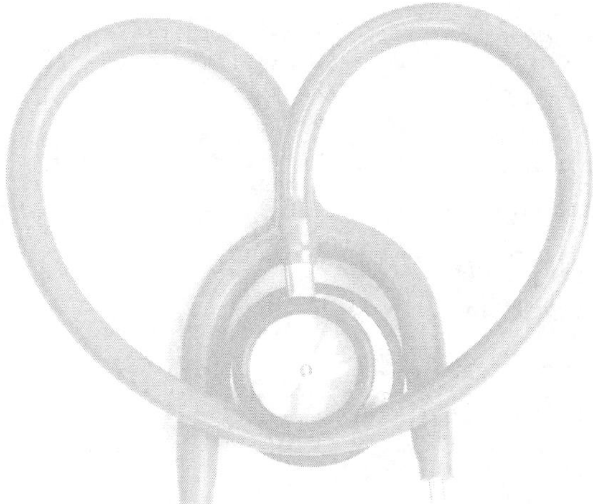

Web Resources

Alateen
www.al-ateen.org

American Academy of Allergy, Asthma, and Immunology
www.aad.org

American Academy of Dermatology
www.aad.org

American Academy of Neurology
www.aan.com

American Academy of Ophthalmology
www.aap.org

American Academy of Pediatrics
www.aao.org

American Association of Kidney Patients
www.aakp.org

American Cancer Society
www.cancer.org

American Heart Association
www.americanheart.com

American Lung Association
www.lungusa.org

Asthma and Allergy Foundation of America
www.aada.org

Centers for Disease Control and Prevention
www.cdc.gov

Cystic Fibrosis Foundation
www.cff.org

Dermatology Foundations
www.dermfnd.org

Emedicine
www.emedicine.com

Harvard Medical School's Consumer Health Information
www.intelihealth.com

Heart Center Online
www.heartcenteronline.com

Hydrocephalus Association
www.hydroassoc.org

Mayo Clinic
www.mayoclinic.com

Narcotics Anonymous
www.na.org

National Asthma Education and Prevention Program
www.nhlbi.nih.gov/about/naepp

National Cancer Institute
www.cancer.gov

National Center for Infectious Disease
www.edc.gov/ncidod

National Center for Learning Disabilities
www.ncld.org

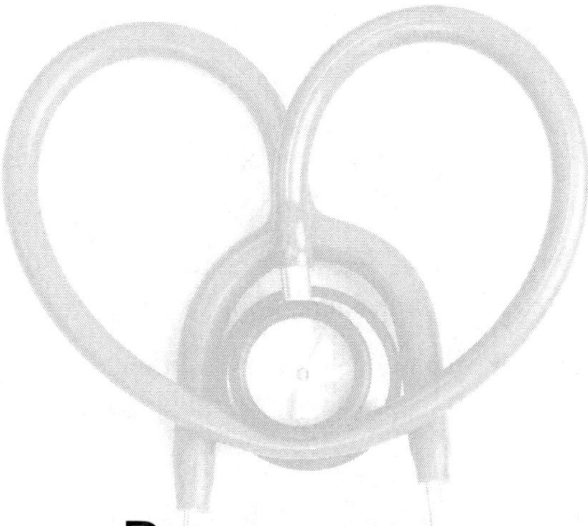

Resources

Bowden, V.R., and Greenberg, C.S. Pediatric Nursing Procedures. Philadelphia: Lippincott Williams & Wilkins, 2003.

Boynton, R.W., et al. Manual of Ambulatory Pediatrics, 5th ed. Philadelphia: Lippincott Williams & Wilkins, 2004.

Engel, J.K. Pocket Guide to Pediatric Assessment, 4th ed. St. Louis: Mosby Year Book Inc., 2002.

Gilbert-Barness, E., and Barness, L.A. Clinical Use of Pediatric Diagnostic Tests. Philadelphia: Lippincott Williams & Wilkins, 2003.

Green-Hernandez, C., et al. Primary Care Pediatrics. Philadelphia: Lippincott Williams & Wilkins, 2001.

Hockenberry, M.J., et al. Wong's Nursing Care of Infants and Children, 7th ed. St. Louis: Mosby Year Book, Inc., 2003.

Hovsepian, Movses. Modell's Current Use and New Drugs. New York: Springer Publishing Co., Inc., 2001.

James, S.R., et. al. Nursing Care of Children: Principles and Practice, 2nd ed. Philadelphia: W.B. Saunders Co., 2002.

Kitchen, WH, et al. Premature Babies: A Guide for Parents. Pennsylvania: Rodale Press, 1985.

Liska, Ken. Drugs and the Human Body: With Implications for Society. New York: Prentice Hall, 2000.

MacArthur, Barton and Anne Dezoete. Early Beginnings: Development in Children Born Preterm. Oxford University Press, 1992.

Mandleco, B. Growth and Development Handbook: Newborn through Adolescent. Clifton Park, N.Y.: Delmar Learning, 2003.

Merck Index: An Encyclopedia of Chemicals, Drugs, and Biologicals. Merck & Company, Inc., 2001.

Merenstein, Gerald B. Handbook of Neonatal Intensive Care. Mosby, 1993.

Muscari, M.E. Advanced Pediatric Clinical Assessment: Skills and Procedures. Philadelphia: Lippincott Williams & Wilkins, 2001.

Pillitteri, A. Maternal and Child Health Nursing: Care of the Childbearing and Childrearing Family, 4th ed. Philadelphia: Lippincott Williams & Wilkins, 2003.

Polin, R.A., and Ditmar, M.F. Pediatric Secrets, 3rd ed. Philadelphia: Hanley & Belfus, 2001.

Rebeschi, L.M., and Brown, M.H. The Pediatric Nurse's Survival Guide, 2nd ed. Clifton Park, N.Y.: Delmar Learning, 2002.

Schwartz, M.W., et al. The 5-minute Pediatric Consult, 3rd ed. Philadelphia: Lippincott Williams & Wilkins, 2003.

Sears, William. Keys to Calming the Fussy Baby. New York: NAL-Dulton, 1996.

Segal, Marilyn. In Time and With Love: Caring for the Special Needs Baby. New York: Newmarket, 1988.

Taketomo, C.K., et al. Pediatric Dosage Handbook, 9th ed. Hudson, Ohio: Lexi-Comp, Inc., 2002.

Zaichkin, Jeanette. Newborn Intensive Care: What Every Parent Needs to Know. Petaluma CA: NICU Ink Book Publishers, 1996. 2004 American Diabetes Association. From Diabetes Care, Vol. 27, Supplement 1, January 2004 Reprinted with permission from The American Diabetes Association.